W9-CPR-007

HOW TO KEEP YOUR YOUTHFUL VITALITY AFTER FORTY

How to Keep Your Youthful Vitality After Forty

by Lelord Kordel

Author of EAT AND GROW YOUNGER

G. P. Putnam's Sons

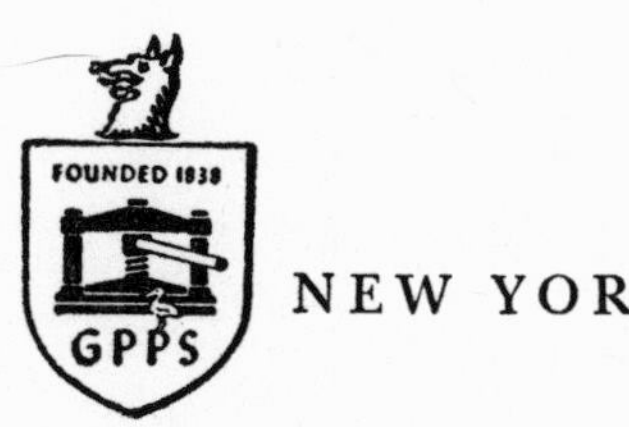

NEW YORK

 Published simultaneously in the Dominion of Canada by Longmans Canada Limited, Toronto.

Library of Congress Catalog Card Number: 77-75586

Printed in the United States of America

Contents

HOW TO KEEP
YOUR YOUTHFUL VITALITY
AFTER FORTY

1

Rogues' Gallery of Rapid Aging

Every person alive is interested in prolonging his life, his mental and physical vigor, and his zest for living. It's as easy as knowing the right foods to eat and the most effective ways of exercising—and preserving the body's natural energies. But before we begin to talk about the ways to a better, longer life, let's first find out how you fit into the picture. Just how badly do you want to live longer?

Never has so much knowledge of health, nutrition and longevity been so available to anyone who will look, listen and read. But you can't help the person who thinks, "Sure, I know all that. Only it doesn't apply to *me*. I'm immune." There is, unfortunately, no immunization against neglect. It takes common sense to recognize it and your own change of attitude and habits to cure it.

The "crimes" people commit are most often against themselves, and their real victims are their loved ones: the wife who must struggle to support the husband who ignored the laws governing his body and was struck down in his prime by a preventable illness; the older woman who sees her husband grow feeble and senile soon after retirement; the widowed mothers and orphaned children. They will all tell you the effect apathy, indifference and neglect have had on their lives.

Nature can be a forgiving mother if we get back in her good graces. But she can be a cruel force if her laws are violated. Perhaps the worst offenders of nature's laws are the smokers and the overeaters. Certainly ignorance of facts is not to blame. Newspapers, magazines, television and radio bombard us with the dangers of excessive smoking. Doctors and scientists have thousands of case histories that reveal the horror of its effects. Yet cigarette sales continue to rise. So do the problems!

Overweight, the other major health hazard, makes you look older, age faster, die younger. In studies of 50,000 overweight people, the Metropolitan Life Insurance Company found that mortality among them was fifty percent higher than average. As weight climbs up to as much as twenty-five percent above normal, the death rate soars to an alarming seventy-five percent.

Faced with this evidence, do the fatties "run scared" from the foods that shorten their lives and decide to do something about their grave condition? (And I *do* mean the kind they are digging!) If they ran scared enough, they wouldn't be fat. Instead, the majority of them continue to stuff themselves at the table. Between meals they raid the refrigerator for leftover cake or pie. And as their waistline gets larger, their lifeline grows shorter.

The list of bad examples could go on and on. But a picture is worth a thousand words. So let's take a look at a few portraits in what might be called our Rogues' Gallery of Rapid Aging.

The Scoffer: This one challenges every known fact with his own theories, which he picks at random out of a grab bag of misinformation. Most of the scoffer's ideas are absolutely worthless. Many are ridiculous. He won't listen to what you have to say. He's too busy trying to convince you he's right and you're wrong.

Sometimes the scoffers try to convince *me*. They come to my lectures not to listen, but to argue. "Vitamins!" one of them said to me. "Who needs them?" Clearly he did. His pudgy body, pasty face, tired, baggy eyes, and confused thinking indicated a high-sugar-and-starch diet that was undoubtedly deficient in essential vitamins, minerals and protein. He had scoffed at the idea that vitamins existed, and at that meeting I had had no chance to convince him otherwise. I never saw him again. But sometimes I wonder how long *he* existed without them.

The Self-Medicator: The scoffer is usually a man. But the self-medicator may be male or female. Self-medicators may disagree on the most effective "cures," but they have one thing in common: They seldom know the meaning of moderation. Some of them are consistent overeaters who try to calm the protests of their overloaded stomachs with bicarbonate of soda and other alkalizers. When these fail to work, they use laxatives and cathartics.

Others—and these are generally women—will tell you that they "don't eat enough to keep a bird alive." This type merely picks at the food set before them. If they live alone, chances are they skip meals entirely. Or they heat a can of soup or macaroni, stir up a prepared no-cook pudding, and consider that a satisfactory dinner. No wonder exhaustion, headaches, insomnia and "nerves" are chronic conditions with them.

A brisk outdoor walk would improve their appetite, but they won't take it. They complain that they are too tired to move. So they sit home drinking coffee, tea and liquor. Or they eat candy in excess. This may give short-lived stimulation, but it doesn't last long enough to drag them out of the easy chair. Their food shelves may be bare, but their medicine chests bulge with a variety of "cures" for all the ailments caused by a starvation diet. The only cure they need is a change to a good diet and better health habits. Tragically, it is a change they refuse to make. So the self-medicators age rapidly as they rely on useless cures. Valuable time is lost—or comes to a final standstill.

The Daredevil: Believes that the phrases "Live dangerously" and "Eat, drink and be merry" were coined for him. He makes a vainglorious effort to live up to them. As a little boy, when bubble gum was scarce, he chewed tar, although he was told it would ruin his teeth. He was the first kid in his school to smoke. And he was always eager to try various cheap and available means of "getting high." Nobody knows why his parents let him get away with it. Maybe they didn't realize that next in line would be liquor, marijuana and LSD trips. So he goes on flying into the face of unnecessary danger with his reckless habits, careless eating and drinking, heavy smoking. He fancies himself a very dashing fellow. But dissipation has lined his face and weakened his body. He has already paid for his childhood addiction to bubble gum, tar and Coke by losing his teeth. Today he wears dentures. And *that* isn't very dashing.

The female daredevil follows much the same pattern as the male. I went to school with one who was a tomboy, proud of her childish record of "always taking a dare." As a teen-ager, she started smoking because somebody dared her, and in college she drank for the same reason. When I saw her last, she was fat, fifty and no longer fair. But she told me, "You know, Lelord, I still can't resist a dare!"

"Haven't you outgrown that yet?" I asked.

"Try me!" she urged, the old daredevil gleam in her eyes. "Dare me to do something."

I did. I made out a diet for her and dared her to lose thirty pounds.

The Procrastinator: "Never do today what you can put off until tomorrow" is his motto. He asks for advice and is grateful for it. But he never follows it. He knows that his habits are hurting his health. He's always going to do something about them . . . tomorrow. *Tomorrow* he'll get up, eat a good breakfast. At night, he continues to reassure himself, he'll go to bed at a decent hour so he can start the next day feeling refreshed. By that time he should be ready for some exercise. So he'll leave the house early and walk part way to work. Maybe he'll join a gym for some workouts.

What does he do, in fact? He goes to the window, takes a deep breath, returns to his desk, then tells his friends how fine he feels on his new health schedule. When they ask how long he's been on it, he answers, "I start tomorrow." But tomorrow never comes. And he goes on procrastinating until it's too late for him to change. Today is the only time we really have to start a new life—or to end one.

The Rebel: A little rebellion is essential to growth and progress. But when resistance and protest become a way of life, they can be dangerous. Even among the young rebels, skipped meals, irregular hours and fatigue take their toll and make them look old for their age. On a recent trip to San Francisco, one of them walked up to me and handed me a flower.

"What's this for?" I asked.

"Man, haven't you heard about us flower children?" he asked in a gentle voice. "Flowers are a symbol. We rebel against hatred and war and go around spreadin' love and goodwill."

He was clean and nonviolent but looked gaunt and hungry. So I invited him to lunch. As we ate, the deep grooves in his face and the thin body that seemed bent with the weight of years prompted me to ask, "Aren't you rather old to be one of the flower children?"

He almost dropped his fork in surprise. "Man, how do you figure? I'm only nineteen."

The middle-aged rebels are probably those that are most in need of help. Yet they are the ones most likely to refuse it. They pride themselves on being nonconformists, yet they are rigidly set in their ways. They hate regimentation, yet their rebellion follows a narrow, inflexible pattern which they refuse to expand or alter. Worst of all, they are against all rules, even those for their own protection. They reject the accepted rules of health and nutrition as ways of improving their health, maintaining their youth and prolonging their lives. Thus, they are in danger of losing all three.

The Fatalist: This person is convinced that his destiny is written in the stars and nothing he can do will change it. He is a wholehearted believer in astrology but ignores the fact that the professional soothsayers admit, "The stars impel; they do not *compel.*"

A fatalist whose mother and sister had died of diabetes complained when I put her on a diet eliminating the sweets she loved. "I don't have diabetes yet," she said, "but I just know that's what will finally kill me. There's nothing I can do about it."

"There's plenty you can do about it," I told her. "You can help prevent it by means within your control. Avoid sweets. Get your weight down to normal. Don't you know the overweight are much more prone to diabetes than those of normal weight?"

"Well, my mother and sister were both fat," she said.

"And they both died young of diabetes," I shot back. "Doesn't that scare you enough to do all you can to prevent it?"

But she had an alibi for that, too. "What I mean is, fat runs in our family. It's my fate to be fat. There's nothing I can do about that either."

"Just how do you think the stars control your destiny?" I asked. "By twinkling down a Morse code message that says, 'Make this one fat; then give her diabetes'? And who carries out the orders? Fate—or *you?*" She went away without taking the diet list I had given her. She would continue gorging on sweets until she became diabetic. Which is just what happened. It took a diabetic coma and a brush with death to change her from a fatalist to a realist. She now controls her own fate—with diet—and the necessary treatments.

These are just a few portraits of the many nominees for early aging and premature death. Some of their stories end with hope for the future. Others have tragic endings that could have been avoided. Which will yours be? Will you recharge your life—or die too soon? The decision is yours to make. But remember what happens to procrastinators. Don't wait too long to make it.

Maybe you don't resemble any of the award winners for aging. So far you've done all right. Youth, luck and heredity have been on your side. Sure, you've taken chances you shouldn't have, yet you've had no disastrous results. *So far.* But if you're forty or past, it's time to quit gambling with your life. Now is the time for a physical inventory. Find out what you've been doing wrong so you can stop it. This book will tell you how to stay alive and youthful during your second forty years. And it may get you to your third forty years. But the results will depend upon your own efforts.

2

How the Mind and Body Grow Old

When and how do we begin to grow old? Just as there are peaks of growth in the human body, so is there a beginning of gradual decline that takes place in each organ. And some of it occurs at a surprisingly early age. By the time a child is in his seventh or eighth year, fat deposits begin to appear on the walls of his aorta, the main artery by which blood leaves the heart. Until recently these changes in the blood vessels were thought to occur only in the aging person. But we also know two vital facts concerning the arteries:

1. The rate of their decline can, to a great extent, be brought under control.
2. Their deterioration can be slowed down *and, in many cases, reversed.*

Other signs of aging also begin early in life. At the age of ten, a child's hearing has reached its peak of keenness. From then on it begins to diminish, so slowly that no change is perceptible for many years. But as he grows older, he gradually loses his ability to hear high-pitched sounds. With advancing age, his hearing may be seriously impaired or lost. Or his loss of hearing may be so slight that the decline goes unnoticed, or almost so, as long as he lives. Before the child is grown, the lens of his eye begins to lose some of its elasticity. Between forty and fifty, he may find that he has trouble focusing without the aid of bifocals.

The male reaches his peak of sexual activity in his teens, after which a slight decline will usually begin to occur. The decline takes place over a long span of years, so slowly that its progress goes unnoticed until the fear of middle age begins. And notice that I said *fear,* since its effects are far more damaging than the results of actual aging. It's a scientific fact that in persons whose physical and emotional health is good, age has little to do with impotence in men or frigidity in women. *The experts are in unanimous agreement that continued sexual performance until late in life depends almost entirely upon two factors: health and attitude.* (This subject and others that are mentioned only briefly here are discussed at length in later chapters.)

A man's muscular strength is at its peak at twenty-five. After his forties, it begins a slow decline. There is some loss of muscle cells, which are not regenerated, as the majority of cells are. Instead, they are replaced by fibrous tissue and fat. Although muscular strength decreases with the passage of time, for some mysterious reason the muscle fiber itself seems to undergo little or no change. If three samples of muscle fiber taken from the muscle of a young man, his father and his grandfather were examined under a microscope, only an expert could see any difference in them. There is reason to believe that the loss of muscular strength may be caused by changes in the chemistry of muscle as we grow older. But more research is needed on it. We know, of course, that poor body chemistry and lack of use will weaken muscles at *any* age.

And at any time of life, from infancy to old age, the process of aging is speeded up by illness and neglect. It sounds easy to say that by preventing illness, avoiding neglect and keeping your mind and body healthy you can stay young longer—but you can! First you have to know how to go about it.

When you stop to consider, you realize that such a project requires the knowledge of experts in a wide variety of subjects. How, you ask, can you be expected to keep up with the latest scientific research in a dozen different fields? Most of you can't. Part of the knowledge this book contains has been gathered from scientists, nutritionists and psychologists from around the world. Part of it is derived from my own lifetime of study and experiments, of searching for the keys to health, youth and longevity. Once you know how to use these keys the results can be transforming.

Many of the things that wreck your health and destroy your youth seem so harmless that you would never suspect them. Your first line of defense is to learn what they are, how and when they are most likely to attack—and how to build up your protection against them. Some of the aging processes are not yet fully understood. This book will tell you which ones have been controlled and those which have not. It will show you how even some of the complex ones are, in different degrees, within your control. You will learn how some of them are not only controllable, but reversible.

But is the loss of strength that occurs over the years an inevitable part of aging? Or is it the cumulative effects of years of neglect and disuse? Many centuries ago these questions were answered by a Roman, Marcus Cato, who during his eighties was still active in the senate, had recently learned Greek, was beginning a serious study of Greek literature—and in his spare time kept busy writing the seventh volume of his *Antiquities*! His answers are just as true today as they were then:

> The loss of muscular strength occurs, but it can be considerably reduced. You should eat to live, not live to eat. Loss of strength is more often chargeable to the dissipations of youth than to any fault of old age, for it delivers to old age a body already worn out.
>
> . . . It is our duty to resist the depredations of age; to compensate for their defects by a watchful care, to fight against them as we would fight against disease; *to adopt a regimen of health; to practice moderate exercise; to take just enough food and drink to restore our strength and not to overburden it.* (My italics)
>
> *Under these conditions the loss of strength, though it cannot be completely prevented, can at least be kept to a minimum.* (My italics)

Since Cato's time, science has made giant strides, but his ideas and our modern expansion of them are still the basic requirements for health, youthful energy and longevity.

Now let's see how the vital organs of the body hold up during an average lifetime.

The Brain

You needn't worry about "using up" your brain. Just the opposite is true. *Not using it enough* can cause mental deterioration. All evidence points to the fact that the brain is a sturdy organ, capable of giving efficient service for the hundred years or more that most authorities on longevity now believe should be the normal human life-span. To function efficiently, the brain requires nourishment, especially protein, lecithin, glutamic acid, B vitamins and vitamins E and D. It must have a *constant supply* of oxygen and sugar (glucose) carried to it by the bloodstream.

Changes within the brain occur very slowly, over a long period of time. The most common causes of mental changes in the elderly do not occur within the brain tissue itself, but rather are caused by hardening of the arteries in the brain (*cerebral arteriosclerosis*). When arteriosclerosis chokes off the brain's source of blood supply, degenerative changes result.

But the mere process of aging is not the cause of senility. If a major artery to the brain is decidely sclerotic, only that part of the brain it supplies will deteriorate. When most of the arteries supplying the brain are affected, *senile dementia* (loss of mental faculties, personality changes, regression, and mental distortions) takes place. A stroke occurs when one of the arteries becomes completely clogged or if it ruptures. (Chapter 15 tells you the best means of preventing hardening of the arteries, of slowing down its progress and, in many cases, reversing it.) Other causes of premature senility are severe illness, physical injury and shock. But just as these conditions improve under proper treatment, so do the mental symptoms triggered by them.

Arteriosclerosis, in varying degrees, remains by far the most common cause of the progressive decline of mental capacities. By preventing it and keeping the arteries unclogged and capable of carrying an adequate supply of blood and other nutrients to the brain, that durable organ will maintain normal function in the healthy person for a long lifetime. But never forget that the active, interested mind that involves itself in learning and in a continuing search for new ideas is the one that retains its youthful outlook. Give it a chance, and the mind can keep on growing as long as you live. Says Dr. Alex Comfort, "We have no final mental stature, as we have a physical stature."

The Liver

If you had a complete failure of liver function, you wouldn't be alive to tell about it. The liver is one of the most important organs in the body, serving as a combination manufacturing plant, chemical laboratory and storehouse of nutrients. It produces and pours into the bloodstream, or stores until needed, many elements the body must have to live. Here are just a few of its functions:

1. The production and storage of substances vital to the manufacture of red blood cells.
2. The elimination of poisons and toxins that circulate throughout the body.
3. Regulation of chemical reactions in the body.
4. The production and storage of protein; the regulation of the numerous byproducts of protein metabolism.
5. The storage of sugar (in the form of glycogen).
6. The storage and utilization of fats.
7. The control of cholesterol metabolism. When liver function is impaired, there is an increase in cholesterol. An early sclerosis of the blood vessels occurs as cholesterol is deposited on their walls.
8. The production of bile acids, bile salts, and substances important for blood coagulation.

As we grow older, there is some destruction of liver cells. But the body has such an excess of liver tissue that unless the loss is extreme, the liver's function is not endangered.

Here's what you can do to keep your liver healthy and its life-sustaining services in good working order:

If you're overweight, reduce. Fatty infiltration of the liver interferes with its function.

Maintain a diet high in nutrients but low in calories. The liver needs plenty of protein, vitamins, and natural sugars obtained from fresh fruits, vegetables, whole grains and honey.

Avoid excessive use of alcohol. Both the chronic alcoholic and the victim of malnutrition have a high incidence of cirrhosis and other liver diseases.

The Kidneys

It used to be a common misconception that a steady decline in kidney function began around the age of forty-five. Only recently has one of the nation's top gerontologists disproved that theory. Dr. Nathan W. Shock and his colleagues have found that *normal kidneys in a healthy person* do not start to deteriorate until very late in life. But note that the emphasis is on *normal* kidneys in a *healthy* person. Severe kidney infections that occur in youth or middle age can lead to premature impairment of kidney function in later years.

The kidneys do undergo some degenerative changes with aging. A portion of the filtering equipment is lost, and hardening of the renal arteries is common in those past sixty who have high blood pressure.

You have already seen how damage to the blood vessels of vital organs can be one of the most serious factors in the aging process. A statistician for the Metropolitan Life Insurance Company, Herbert H. Marks, gives us these facts on the mortality rate: "Fifty-five percent of the money paid out in death claims in one year by the Metropolitan was accounted for *by diseases of the blood vessels in the heart, brain, or kidneys.*" (My italics)

When the kidneys' tiny arteries harden or are blocked by fatty deposits, it decreases the supply of blood they receive, prevents the nutrients from being reabsorbed and inhibits the excretion of highly toxic urea, a condition that can cause fatal uremic poisoning.

Destroyed kidney tissue does not regenerate. But just as the body has extra liver tissue, it also contains a surplus of kidney tissue. The body can lose as much as three-fourths of its total amount of kidney tissue and still maintain adequate function. There is no evidence that the removal of one kidney shortens the life-span—*as long as the remaining kidney is healthy and continues to perform satisfactorily.*

One of the kidneys' indispensable functions is to prevent the loss from the bloodstream of essential chemicals and substances needed to maintain normal body chemistry. Another is to filter the blood and extract from it the accumulation of poisons, waste and excess minerals and water. An adult has about 6 quarts of blood in his body. But due to the continuous circulation of blood, the kidneys have the colossal task of filtering approximately 5,500 quarts a day! If the kidneys fail to function adequately, degeneration of other organs results, and the life-span is shortened. When a complete kidney failure occurs, death follows rapidly.

Some Major Causes of Kidney Damage

1. Hardening of the small arteries (arterioles) in the kidneys and of the arteries going to the kidneys. (See Chapter 15 for preventive suggestions that include lecithin, magnesium, vitamin E and the B vitamins, especially choline, inositol and B_6.)
2. Undernourishment, with inadequate maintenance of protein levels in the body.
3. Marked anemia, which results in an insufficient supply of blood and oxygen. To give your kidneys the large amounts of blood rich in oxygen they require, eat foods rich in blood-building iron. (See Chapter 5.)
4. Kidney infection of bacterial origin.
5. Blockage of the kidney exit caused by kidney stones.
6. In men, blockage because of an enlarged prostate gland.

7. Poisoning from certain toxins that circulate in the bloodstream, or from some drugs, particularly those containing mercury.

8. Occasionally one of the antibiotics used to treat infections or an overdose of some medication that would otherwise be harmless.

The Pancreas

This important gland and its vital functions are discussed at length in a later chapter. (The heart and arteries are also covered in separate chapters.)

The Lungs

The lungs hold up remarkably well under the aging process. They have such a tremendous reserve power that about half the lung tissue has to be damaged or destroyed before serious symptoms develop.

Experiments have shown that age has no effect on the circulation of blood through the lungs. Pressure tests and oxygen tests made by Dr. Lewis Dexter and his associates at Harvard Medical School and the Peter Bent Brigham Hospital showed little or no difference in pulmonary circulaton between the young and the aged. Their report stated: "There is an enormous pulmonary vascular reserve, so the cross-sectional area of the pulmonary vasculature (vessels) *must be reduced more than half before changes in circulation or flow through the lungs can be detected.*" (My italics)

There is a gradual loss of elastic tissue in the lungs of an aging person, but according to a British pathologist, Dr. Donald Heath, it begins early in life and is not a direct result of the aging process. Dr. Heath, a senior lecturer in pathology at the University of Birmingham in England, explains that "while this condition is found in the elderly . . . these changes occur at about the age of twenty and progress steadily throughout adult life."

This does not mean that no degenerative changes take place in the aging lungs. The walls of the air cells tend to break down, and some of the elastic tissue is replaced by fibrous tissue. Both of these processes lessen the capacity of the lungs to extract oxygen from the air. *But the effects of the aging process on the lungs are slight compared to the damage caused by other controllable factors.* Air pollution, untreated or chronic respiratory infections and *especially cigarette smoking* have caused an alarming rise in emphysema, pulmonary fibrosis (scarring of the lungs), and lung cancer. Here are some recommended ways of protecting yourself from these dangers:

1. STOP SMOKING! If you can't stop, or think you can't, at least cut down as much as possible, avoid deep inhalation and see Chapter 11 for protective measures against the ravages of lung cancer.
2. Keep home and office well ventilated and free of smoke and stale air.
3. Whenever possible, avoid inhalation of dust, fumes, chemicals and other sources of air pollution.
4. Do all you can to prevent respiratory infections. (Add vitamins A and C complex, rich in the bioflavonoids, to a well-balanced diet.)
5. Any symptom of a bacterial or viral infection should have immediate treatment to avoid a chronic condition.

The Adrenals

The two tiny tricorn-shaped glands that rest astride each kidney are called our fight-or-flight glands, or our glands of survival. The hormones produced and secreted by these small glands are so indispensable to life that if a total failure of adrenal activity occurred, death would soon follow.

Each gland is divided into two parts: the outer "shell," called the *cortex,* and the *medulla,* or center. The cortex is vital to the regulation of blood pressure, kidney function and muscular power. No less than twenty-eight compounds have been isolated from the cortex, with the most spectacular one, cortisone, deriving its name from it. Other essential functions performed by the cortex are:

1. The secretion of certain male and female hormones. (In the case of decreased secretions of sex hormones, the adrenals will secrete their own sex hormones.)

2. The production of chemicals that strengthen the body's resistance to infection, toxins, injury and stress.

3. The utilization of virtually all blood chemistry in the tissues.

4. The regulation of the body's balance of carbohydrates, salt, water and minerals.

A comparatively rare but usually fatal illness, Addison's disease, results from an underactivity of the adrenal cortex. Glaucoma, a major cause of blindness, has been found to occur with adrenal exhaustion. Other results of adrenal underactivity are allergies, faulty mineral metabolism, and such symptoms associated with old age as generalized weakness, low metabolism, slow reactions, extreme mental and physical fatigue and decreased sexual capacity. The failure of the cortex to produce sufficient cortisone is believed to be a primary factor in the onset of arthritis. Plenty of vitamin C added to a balanced diet increases the production and utilization of cortisone and aids the antibiotic function of the cortex. The adrenals are the first of the glands to be damaged by a deficiency of protein, B vitamins (especially pantothenic acid), vitamin C and linoleic acid.

The symptoms of an overactive cortex include so many deviations from the normal that those affecting sexuality are grouped together under the medical name *andreno-genital syndrome*. You may have seen some of the victims of this syndrome in circus sideshows as the Bearded Lady, the Man Who Turned into a Woman (or vice versa) and assorted specimens of the Third Sex. Another condition caused by overactivity of the cortex is called Cushing's disease. The victim of this disfiguring malady has such an excessive amount of fat deposited around the neck and shoulders that he resembles a buffalo.

The adrenal medulla produces and secretes *epinephrine* and *norepinephrine*, better known as adrenalin and noradrenalin.

Adrenalin is your fight-or-flight hormone. It supplies the body with immediate and supernormal strength in response to an emergency situation by feeding the heart with fast-burning glucose, alerting the brain, quickening the reflexes and strengthening the muscles. The medical value of adrenalin is well known. It acts with dramatic speed to relieve the person suffering from a severe attack of allergy, the asthmatic patient gasping for breath, and in countless life-and-death crises of heart failure.

Endocrinologist Dr. Herman H. Rubia, author of several books about the glands, says that "perhaps the familiar line, 'a man is as old as his arteries,' will be replaced by 'a man is as old as his adrenals!' " Certainly there are many researchers who believe that the aging process itself is brought on, or at least accelerated, by a decrease in adrenal function. You can help prevent that decrease! The evidence all points to the fact that adrenal function can be maintained at normal levels in the older person—*as long as his health is good.*

The vital organs that hold the key to health and longevity have enough reserve to keep you well and vigorous for a lifetime. Your body is an efficient, self-renewing organism. Give it the nourishment, the activity and the rest it needs to regenerate itself. Your mind has no final stature. Keep it alert, interested and growing, and it will continue to develop its active, productive powers. You must also avoid the damaging forms of neglect and abuse that can destroy your health of mind and body. If you don't, they can condemn you to illness, premature old age and an untimely death. The choice is yours.

You can also control the rate at which your body ages. In the next chapter we will see how you can retard the aging process by simple changes in your attitudes, diet and amount of activity.

3

What Determines Your Rate of Aging?

Biochemists, nutritionists and psychologists from all parts of the world offer varying observations and explanations of what controls the aging process.

"You are as young as your arteries." This classic statement is credited to Canada's widely quoted Dr. William Osler. Clogged, hardened arteries *can* cause premature aging, illness and death.

"You are as young as your connective tissues," according to Russia's noted scientist Dr. Alexander A. Bogomolets, who insists that, "A man of sixty or seventy is still young. He has lived only half his natural life."

"You are as young as your colon," averred another Russian, bacteriologist Elie Metchnikoff, in his world-famous book on the subject, *The Prolongation of Life.* He recommended acidophilus buttermilk and yogurt to keep the colon healthy. These milk products produce "friendly" bacteria in the intestinal tract, which combat the toxins released by decomposing food and which Dr. Metchnikoff believed are the primary cause of aging.

From France comes another opinion, also backed by verified facts. In his book, *Prolonger la Vie,* Dr. Saint-Pierre wrote, "You are as young as your blood." With a vast amount of evidence to substantiate it, endocrinologists tell us that we are as young as our glands. Psychologists have thousands of case histories to prove that we are as young as our minds. And from Stockholm, Sweden, cames this comment of a prominent doctor: "Every individual grows old on his own pattern," says Dr. F. Henschen. ". . . People must learn that inactivity accelerates the aging process and that *activity* preserves physical and psychological health."

There is truth in all of these statements. But not the whole truth. Each of the doctors and scientists quoted spoke in terms of his own specialized knowledge. But to benefit most from that knowledge, we must combine all their areas of research. We must expand those areas as we go along. We must take advantage of the newest discoveries that are continually being made. And finally, we must know how to put this knowledge to practical use. The *total* body and mind can *resist* premature aging if it is kept strong and healthy. It is a lifetime project. And the sooner you start, the better. But don't attempt it all at once. Take it in progressive steps, chapter by chapter, one problem at a time, as we intend to do.

Some of the problems of premature aging may be unique. But the majority of them are universal, things that have happened, will happen or *could* happen to you. You may be as old as clogged arteries, as an impoverished bloodstream, as an unhealthy colon, as starved cells or tissues due to a poorly nourished body. You may be as old as a morbid, suspicious attitude. Or your age may be measured by a mind that is closed and rusting from lack of use. Maybe your mind doesn't creak but your joints do. And, through neglect, perhaps your muscles have grown too weak to hold you erect.

Our goal must be the health of the body *and* mind as a *whole,* not just parts of it. Dr. Hans Selye, famous for his research on stress, put it this way: "Life, the biologic chain that holds our parts together, is only as strong as its weakest link. When this breaks, no matter which vital link it may be—our parts can no longer be held together as a single living being."

We shall see how three factors—nutrition, activity, and mental outlook—are the most important elements in determining the condition of our bodies and often the length of our lives. Whatever your "weak links," you will learn from the actual cases in this book what you can do to help yourself.

Your entire body, from your heart to your brain, from your cells and tissues to your bloodstream, depends for survival upon the food you eat. *Nutrition,* therefore, is the foundation for any program designed to help you stay young longer. Knowing *what* to eat is important. But you must also know what *not* to eat. Dr. Selye suggested that aging may be caused partly by an accumulation of waste products that prevent the cells from receiving their proper nourishment. There are foods that contribute to this condition by clogging up the body's machinery. They starve your cells, brain, glands and other organs of vital nutrients. These "empty foods" weaken the different links of your "biologic chain" by causing degenerative damage. In its advanced stages, this damage becomes almost impossible to repair and reverse.

But you can help yourself by keeping your own bloodstream healthy. There is nothing more involved than the time required to keep the blood circulating briskly and no extra cost beyond that of the food you eat—if that food is wisely chosen. When properly nourished, each cell in the body is capable of building its own resistance. And with the exception of nerve and brain cells, each cell has an almost miraculous power to reproduce itself.

Your rate of aging depends upon whether or not these cells function normally. They *cannot* function normally unless you give them the proper nourishment.

How many of the so-called middle-aged crises—
the cycle of anxieties and depression,
the physical aches and pains,
the bleak mental attitude,
the loss of looks with early wrinkling, and
the decline of energy and virility or femininity—
are directly traceable to deficiencies that are caused, not by age, but by years of poor nutritional habits?

When the body is starved of protective food elements, it tires and ages rapidly. The mind loses its alertness, is less able to concentrate, and emotional difficulties become harder to deal with. These difficulties range from mild depression to inability to cope with reality. Assorted instabilities, fears and inadequacies develop that can make living a nightmare.

Nutrition must be the basis of any program designed to help you stay young longer. Ideally, a diet should supply the nutritional needs of all parts of your body *over and above normal requirements.* It must also leave a margin of safety to allow for inadequate absorption in cases of illness and deficiencies. As metabolism slows down, it is wise to reinforce our meals with supplements that are potent in food value but low in calories. (See Chapter 17, "Food Supplements for Your Second Forty Years.")

Activity is another essential of a long, youthful life, not only physical activity to keep the muscles firm and strong, but activity of the mind, to keep thought processes and emotions flexible, responsive, perceptive. By making activity an integral part of life, you will avoid a familiar form of stagnation, with its concomitant, early aging.

Your mental attitude, the way you habitually look at life, can also delay or accelerate your rate of aging. The best way to start coasting downhill by the time you're forty is to expect to do so. Don't! A "what's the use" attitude can age you much faster than if you *think* and *feel* young. Bernard Baruch, when he was past eighty, said, "I always think of old age as being fifteen years older than I am."

All of these considerations add up to the fact that your rate of aging depends upon *you,* upon your pattern of living, what you eat, your daily activities, what you think and feel, the interaction and coordination of your body, mind and emotions. These form your pattern of aging. If the pattern is bad, it can be changed. But you must know what to do and how to do it. And you must do it *now.*

4

Begin Now to Look and Feel Younger!

British playwright Harold Pinter, during the run of his twelfth play, *The Homecoming,* told an interviewer, "I feel pretty exhausted now that I'm thirty-six." He is a victim of chronic exhaustion, also known as pooped-out-itis. Pinter expressed it best when he said, "Dragging yourself around day after day is a hell of a burden."

Chronic exhaustion is brought on not by aging, but by neglect, and is well on the increase. People involved in manual work have temporary bouts with it. But their constant physical activity, generally healthy appetites and the ability to relax after muscular exertion prevent it from reaching the chronic stage. Otherwise, exhaustion isn't choosy about its victims. From childhood on, no one group is immune. It claims people from the ranks of students, office workers, professional men and women, housewives–regardless of age.

Chronic exhaustion is to be distinguished from "fortyitis," which is the *phobia* of oncoming age and gradual decline. Forty as the arbitrary dividing line between youth and age exists only in the minds of those who fear it. I have consulted experts in geriatrics (the science of aging) in Australia, England, France and the United States. In each country I interviewed hundreds of persons of all ages. Some were under thirty and already showing signs of premature aging—signs that are *preventable* and *reversible.* Others, more than twice as old, retained a youthful body, mind and spirit.

The complaints that I heard most often, with shocking regularity even among the young, were these:

"Always tired."

"Pooped out."

"Can't sleep . . . wake up dopey."

"Jumpy nerves . . . can't relax."

"Headaches . . . heartburn."

"Irritable . . . tense . . . anxious."

"Tired."

"Nervous stomach . . . indigestion."

"Flabby muscles . . . stiff joints . . . aching back."

"Overweight . . . potbelly . . . decline of potency."

"Tired . . . *tired* . . . t-i-r-e-d . . ."

If any of these apply to you, don't blame your age. Fortyitis and pooped-out-itis are not synonymous. The burden of dragging yourself around is *not* an inevitable part of growing older. Neglect, not age, is the real culprit. Chronic fatigue, the most constant lament in nearly every age group, can make you look and feel older than you are. So will the other common complaints. Yet all of them are preventable. Or, if it's too late to prevent them they can, in the majority of cases, be corrected—whether you're under thirty or over eighty.

"Neglect myself? Not me!" A forty-year-old friend of mine, Don Braden, was vehement in his denial. "When I saw I was getting a paunch, I went right out and bought an electric vibrator belt."

"How did it work?" I asked, looking at his potbelly.

"So far, not so good," he admitted. "I think there's a little defect in its mechanism."

"In *whose* mechanism?" I asked.

To help Don reduce, I planned a health regime for him. Investigating his eating habits, I learned that coffee and cigarettes were all he had for breakfast. "To keep my weight down," he explained. But this defeats his purpose. By midmorning, he's hungry and irritable. Concentration becomes difficult. Fatigue catches up with him, and he slumps mentally and physically under the burden. So he has a sweet roll and more coffee for "quick energy." An hour or two later, a few martinis chase away the recurring exhaustion. The rest of the day and evening he continues to load up on high-starch foods and high-calorie drinks. Then, overfed but undernourished, he hopes massage will reduce his potbelly.

He chain-smokes because he's nervous. He drinks because he's exhausted. He takes sleeping pills because he can't sleep, pep pills to wake him up, and tranquilizers to relieve tension. He gulps an assortment of fizz powders and tablets for everything from headaches to indigestion. And he calls all this "taking care of myself"!

What *is* the price of health, and a longer, lasting youth? It's very little indeed! It's the price of meat, eggs, fish, poultry, fresh fruits and vegetables. Compare this cost with dozens of boxes of pills and doctor bills. And the pounds of coffee, cigarettes and liquor that too often take the place of regular meals. Many sources of vitality are free. A walk costs nothing. Neither does exercise. Yet both will tone your muscles, aid glandular activity, step up circulation and give you a glow of well-being.

Dr. Tom Spies, one of the great nutritionists of our time, stated at a meeting of the American Medical Association a few years ago that by keeping our bodies in chemical balance through proper nutrition *we can make old age wait.* "As tissues become damaged because they lack the chemicals of good nutrition, they tend to become old," he said. ". . . There are people of forty whose brains and arteries are senile . . ." This early and unnatural breakdown of the mind and body is caused by what scientists call *internal chemical starvation* and *cumulative nutritional deficiencies.* In other words, years of poor eating habits are to blame. And you yourself are responsible for them.

The chronic exhaustion mentioned by Harold Pinter is not, as he seems to think, the result of his thirty-six years. Later in the conversation, he accidentally revealed the real reason for it.

"This morning I was up at nine thirty," he said, "and had grapefruit and a cup of tea." I'm very much in favor of fruit for breakfast, lunch or dinner. I recommend it to start a meal, to end a meal, or between meals. The only time I *don't* advise it is as a substitute for a complete meal that should be built around protein.

Now let's find out how a man more than twice Pinter's age has managed to retain the almost cyclonic energy that, along with his famous nose, has been his trademark during fifty-seven years in show business. Jimmy Durante, at seventy-five, thrives on a heavy schedule. Between television performances, he took the time to tell how he did it. "I can't keep goin' without my health," Jimmy said. "You gotta stay healthy to have energy, and you gotta eat right to stay healthy. I watch my diet—only eat broiled meats and fresh stuff. No gravy, fancy sauces or rich creamed junk to clog up the old machinery."

On avoiding tensions and pressures, he said, "Tension is an energy grabber, so you gotta relax and not get nervous when things go wrong. Look at Jack Benny, how relaxed he is—and Maurice Chevalier, past eighty and still goin' strong—both of 'em with as much pep as ever." On longevity, he had two words of advice, "Stay alive!" How to stay alive was also summed up in two words, "Stay healthy!" And the way to do that: "Like I already said, you gotta eat right to stay healthy, and my old stomach tells me right away when I slip."

Asked about his retirement, Jimmy said, "Me quit? Whatta you want me to do, dry up and blow away? Let 'em stop da music—but not me!" With his genius for mispronouncing words, Jimmy probably couldn't say "cumulative nutritional deficiences," but he doesn't need to say it. He does better than that. He avoids them.

There is no time in your life, from youth to old age, when you cannot benefit by the four rules that Jimmy follows instinctively:

1. "Good eatin' habits." A diet that supplies all the needs of your body.

2. Physical activity. The type best suited to your age and way of life.

3. Mental activity. Having a variety of interests promotes a youthful, optimistic mental outlook.

4. The ability to relax.

"But how can I be sure when a diet supplies all my needs," some people may ask. "And how can I tell what those needs are?" You can start by taking a long, honest look at the body you live in, at the mind that controls it, and at your daily habits. Then decide for yourself, or with some outside help, whether they are working for you or against you.

But the big question is still *how*. "*How* do I know what to do about my needs after I know what they are?" "*How* can I recognize the pitfalls that lead to rapid aging?" "*How* can I avoid nutritional deficiencies?" "*How* do I eat properly?"

Because of individual variances in body chemistry, there can be a vast difference in the way we absorb our food. For one person, "eating properly" may mean just that. For another, because of faulty absorption, it can mean an invitation to multiple deficiencies and rapid aging. In the pages ahead you will learn just what foods are necessary to prevent and correct major and minor deficiencies, to keep the tissues of your vital organs healthy, to renew your cells, to give your endocrine glands the nutrients they must have if they are to supply you with their youth-prolonging hormone secretions. And that's only the beginning. Scientists, nutritionists and psychologists have, in their separate fields, discovered methods that can be used singly or in combination to delay the onset of old age, to combat and in many cases reverse the premature aging that already exists.

For centuries men have searched in vain for the fountain of youth. It may well be that the search is almost over and that the long-sought goals will become a reality within our lifetime. The promise that such a future holds for you—if you follow the rules of a sound health regimen—is a long, youthful life free from the infirmities of age. In the next chapter we will consider the first and most important factor in a lifetime regimen for good health.

5

Protein—the Basis of Life and Youth

Almost 130 years ago, a chemist isolated a substance he claimed was the basis of life. This primary substance was named *protein,* from the Greek word meaning "to come first." Protein is the basis of life, the building material of which all living tissues are made. It is the *only* food substance that can repair and rebuild cells. It is therefore a life-giving substance, a health restorer and a life prolonger.

Protein is also used in making antibodies, without which the body would be powerless to fight off the viruses and toxins that continually invade it. *Experiments have shown that within a week on a high-protein diet, the body's production of antibodies increases as much as 100 times than when fed on meals low in protein.*

The experience of Iris Graham, a thin-faced, undernourished girl who once came to me for some much-needed advice, is typical of people who exist on a low-protein diet.

"I'm really very diet-conscious," she insisted.

"Do you mean *diet*-conscious or nutrition-conscious?" I asked. "There's a big difference."

She had come to this first interview with a vicious cold. As she stared at me over her handkerchief, she complained, "I get one cold after another, even though I eat salads and drink orange juice."

"That's a good start," I said, "but it isn't enough. You need plenty of the protective foods to build up your resistance. During an infection, you should take additional supplements of vitamin C. This aids protein in forming antibodies. *But protein is the first and most important of the protective foods."*

I didn't need to ask what she ate for breakfast and luncheon. She told me later, and it was just what I suspected: orange juice, toast and tea for breakfast, a salad at noon. Dinner, which she often skipped, supplied her with the only complete protein of the day. But not enough of it! Less than a fourth of what she should have!

The beginning of premature aging was already showing in this young girl's face and body. She was a good example of what Dr. Charles S. Davidson of Harvard Medical School affirms, *that most of the symptoms attributed to old age, which include tiring easily and the early sagging, withering and wrinkling of the skin, are due mainly to a protein deficiency.* I've seen the effects of it in the shrunken, wizened faces of tiny children in undeveloped countries. Substandard diets dangerously low in protein drastically shorten their lives.

But Iris Graham lived in England, where plenty of meat, fish, poultry, dairy products were available. During hundreds of interviews I found a shocking number of other young persons who were already showing signs of premature aging.

Iris Graham's symptoms of the deficiences that cause early aging were due to a lack of knowledge concerning the essentials of nutrition. I put her on a high-protein diet to build up her resistance, while keeping her slender but firm. The premature aging of her body had to be reversed! She learned that *protein foods, with their specific dynamic action, are thirty-five percent less fattening than starches and fats.* Moreover, "when diets contain ample protein," according to the U.S. Department of Agriculture Yearbook (1959), "the body can store some of it in the tissues to use in emergencies . . . The day's meals should provide enough protein to meet the body's needs for maintaining and repairing all of its substances and to provide for building reserves of body protein in its tissues."

"Protein," I told Iris, "helps keep your muscles firm and strong, your skin smooth and elastic and your facial contours youthful."

"I never thought I was old enough to worry about that," Iris said, "but I've noticed lately, especially when I'm tired, that my face looks as though it would collapse if a door slammed."

"A low-protein diet hastens aging at *any* age," I told her, "but you can reverse your signs of premature aging by building each of your meals around protein foods." I gave Iris this little chart as an easy way of remembering the protein foods she needed and where to find them:

1. In living tissue: meat, poultry and fish.
2. In food meant to nourish newborn life: milk (also cheese, yogurt and other milk products) and eggs.
3. In seeds of plants in their natural state (not refined or chemically treated): cereal and seed grains (millet and sunflower seeds are particularly good sources of high-grade vegetable protein), nuts and legumes, especially soybeans, which are a complete vegetable protein.

The Importance of Amino Acids

The protein you eat can't be used by your body until it has been broken down by digestive processes into its separate amino acids. Amino acids are simply the *traveling* form of protein that journeys through your bloodstream, reconstructed by that master builder, your body, into the hundreds of varieties of body protein that can be used by many different types of cells. The cells then choose the amino acids they need to repair or replace those that are worn out, and to construct new body tissue, enzymes, antibodies, hormones and other vital substances that need renewing.

Whether you're young or old, you need protein every day of your life. If your meals provide more than enough for your immediate needs, your liver takes amino acids from your bloodstream and stores them until the cells need a new supply. *You age faster on the days that you don't eat enough protein to meet your body's needs.*

The stored supply of protein can be drawn on as long as it lasts. But when it's used up without being replenished—or if you didn't have any stored—the less important body cells are consumed to free amino acids that are necessary to repair or replace those with more vital functions. Skin cells are among the less vital ones that soon show effects of protein deficiency. As hormone secretions diminish, the skin loses its moisture. Membranes dry and shrivel. Muscles grow slack. Sagging begins and wrinkles form prematurely.

If your doctor tells you that you're "out of nitrogen balance," that means you haven't been eating enough of the foods that provide essential amino acids. This can bring about serious deficiencies that will make you age faster than you should. It isn't necessary for you to know the hard-to-remember names of the amino acids. The important thing is to remember the foods that contain them and to make a habit of eating them! But if you'd like to be on speaking terms with the essential ten, here they are:

Arginine	Methionine
Histidine	Phenylalanine
Isoleucine	Threonine
Leucine	Tryptophane
Lysine	Valine

Their valuable functions include not only repairing tissues, but helping to protect you from nervous disorders, digestive trouble, hardening of the liver, nephritis, incipient anemia, respiratory disorders, and many other diseases, in addition to such dreaded signs of aging as losing control of muscular movements, sex gland deterioration and loss of sexual desire and ability.

Some nutritionists list only eight of the amino acids as essential, omitting arginine and histidine. The reason for this is that while the body can manufacture these two, it does so very slowly, especially during periods of stress. Histidine is needed to repair cells and produce normal blood supplies. When arginine (called the fatherhood amino acid) is lacking, sexual instincts and ability decrease in both men and women.

Others may quibble over a technicality, but as long as there is a health hazard involved (for either young or old), I'll hold to my opinion that there are not eight, but ten essential amino acids, including arginine and histidine. These two important amino acids can be provided abundantly and rapidly with the other eight in meals built around the complete proteins.

You need enough each day to meet the body's needs, for maintenance, repair, renewal, and to build a reserve supply of body protein (amino acids) in the tissues. But, even with adequate absorption and no deficiencies, your need for protein may be much greater than the average. Increased tensions and pressures create a need for more protein, as do sudden stresses, shock, illness, accidents and injuries.

A few years ago the Food and Nutrition Board of the National Research Council recommended 60 grams of protein a day for women (85 to 100 grams during pregnancy and lactation), and 70 grams for men. But in a world of ever-mounting tensions and in the light of newer nutritional knowledge, the majority of researchers today advise 100 to 150 grams daily for all adults, with *at least* half of this protein derived from animal sources whenever possible.

Listed below are sources of the most biologically active animal proteins with the approximate protein content of an average serving (usually estimated at about 1/4 pound):

HIGHEST QUALITY ANIMAL PROTEINS

Meat and Poultry	*Amount*	*Approx. Grams Protein*
Beef, lean (rib, rump, pot roast)	1 serving	22
Brains, beef	2 med. pieces	10
Chicken	1 serving	23
Duck	1 serving	20
Goose	1 serving	21
Heart, beef	1 serving	19

Kidney, beef or lamb	1 serving	19
Lamb roast	1 serving	23
Lamb chops	2 average	20
Liver, calf, beef or lamb	1 serving	23
Liver, chicken	1 serving	26
Steak	1 serving	21
Sweetbreads	½ cup	14
Tongue, beef	3 slices	22
Turkey	1 serving	22
Veal, roast leg	1 serving	20
Veal chops	1 serving	18
Veal cutlets	1 serving	19

Fish and Seafood	*Amount*	*Approx. Grams Protein*
Anchovies	6 filets	10
Clams	6	14
Codfish	1 serving	16
Crabmeat	⅔ cup	16
Haddock	1 serving	18
Halibut	1 serving	19
Herring	1 medium	19
Lobster	1 serving	19
Oysters	7 medium	12
Salmon, canned	½ cup	22
Sardines	6 average	13
Scallops	4–5 average	16
Shad	1 serving	19
Shad roe	1 serving	12
Shrimp	6 medium	8
Tuna, canned	⅓ cup	12
Whitefish	1 serving	22

(Other varieties of freshwater fish average about 19 to 21 grams of protein per serving.)

Dairy Products	*Amount*	*Approx. Grams Protein*
Buttermilk	1 quart	30
Cheese, cheddar	2 x 1 x 1	12
" cottage	½ cup	20
" Italian, grated	2 tbsp.	12
" Swiss	2 x 1 x 1	12
Eggs	1 medium	6
Milk, powdered skim	½ cup, level	20
Milk, whole or skim	1 quart	34
Yogurt	1 quart	34

These are complete protein foods containing all of the essential amino acids. The meat, poultry and fish group provides the most concentrated source of biologically active protein since *animal proteins most closely resemble the protein of your body.*

These protein foods supply a maximum amount of usable body protein in relation to the amount eaten. It is wise to keep in mind that the cheaper cuts of meat are just as good—and sometimes better in terms of nutrition—than expensive steaks and chops. Variety and organ meats are budget-priced, yet they are highest of all in amino acids and other nutritive factors.

Here are the minimum protein requirements I have been advocating for years:

At least two daily servings per person from the meat group of foods (including organ meats two or three times a week) *or* substitutions from the poultry or fish group.

And each day:

A choice of foods from the dairy group, including a pint or more of buttermilk, skim milk, yogurt, cottage cheese, or their equivalent. Eggs and milk products are complete animal proteins of high quality, but except for cottage cheese (twenty grams in an average serving), they contain at most only about half the amount of protein per serving as meat, poultry or fish.

Use the dairy foods to supplement other meals. Have eggs, cheese, yogurt, buttermilk, or nonfat milk for between-meal snacks. They are excellent as protein boosters and do double duty by supplying a big share of your calcium needs. When you want to substitute dairy products for the more biologically active proteins, combine several of them at a meal. An omelette, of course, uses eggs, milk and cheese. The use of skim milk powder here can be very rewarding.

To these foods can be added green salads, and green and yellow vegetables, as many raw as possible. Fresh fruits are the best desserts—and only an occasional "dissipation" should be permitted. For faster rehabilitation, I suggest some of the complete and highly concentrated vegetable proteins that you'll be hearing more about in a later chapter.

Here are five basic rules of the plan that worked so well for Iris she gave it this name:

"Rejuvenation Regimen"

RULE 1: *Plenty of high-grade protein each day.* Iris had a wide choice from the groups already mentioned. *Meat, poultry or fish.* A minimum of two daily servings. Liver two or three times a week.

Dairy products: Buttermilk, yogurt, cottage cheese or skim milk (made protein-rich by adding some powdered skim milk), one pint or more a day. Natural, unprocessed cheese as desired.

Eggs: About ten a week, cooked to individual taste.

Bread and cereal: Whole grain only. (Millet meal, available in health food stores, makes an excellent cereal, high in protein and other nutrients.) Breads and cereals should be used with discretion—don't overdo.

Seeds and nuts: In salads, desserts, as snacks and nibbles to boost your protein intake. Highest in protein are sunflower seeds, peanuts, almonds, walnuts.

Legumes, dried: Two or three servings a week, as desired. Soybeans are especially valuable as they contain high-quality protein that can substitute for meat.

Protein supplements: Brewer's yeast and wheat germ were the two that helped Iris in her dramatic recovery. Twice a day usually midmorning and midafternoon, when her energy ebbed, she dissolved two to four tablespoons of brewer's yeast in tomato or vegetable juice. When she ate cereal, she added one-half cup of wheat germ to it.

RULE 2: *An abundance of vitamins and minerals.* A minimum of three or four servings of vegetables each day. Include raw leafy salad greens, tomatoes, yellow and green vegetables and other varieties in season. Choice of two or more fresh raw fruits, melon or berries each day.

RULE 3: *Enzymes are a daily essential.* Cooking kills enzymes. This is one of the reasons I advise raw fruits and vegetables as often as possible. Until recently it was believed enzymes were obtainable only in raw fruits and vegetables. Now we know of a few other potent foods that supply them. See Chapter 10 for more about these little-known, but highly essential substances.

RULE 4: *Avoid devitalized carbohydrates.* Limit your sugars and starches to natural carbohydrates. These are found in fresh fruits and vegetables, whole grains and seed cereals. Instead of refined white sugar, use the more healthful sweeteners as honey, molasses, unrefined raw sugar.

RULE 5: *Eat desserts that provide health dividends.* Choose from any of these:

Protein-rich desserts: Baked custard, junket, sherbet (made with milk or yogurt and fruit). Bavarians (combinations of gelatin, fruit and milk or yogurt). Nuts. Natural, unprocessed cheeses.

Vitamin-and-mineral-rich desserts: Fresh fruits, melons and berries. Eat them plain or with yogurt or cheese.

Occasional substitutes: Dried unsulphured fruits, soaked to tenderness or lightly cooked. Sweeten with honey if desired.

All-time substitutes: To satisfy a craving for candy or cake, reach for the natural, mineral-rich sweetness to be found in dates, figs, raisins, bananas.

There are no magic formulas or drugs that will restore the damage already caused by neglect and that will keep you young all your life. But there is a nutritional plan based on wholesome, everyday foods and supplements that can work seeming miracles in helping you retain your health, youthful appearance and positive mental outlook.

For optimum health, it is also important to know and protect yourself from the deficiencies that slowly but surely ravage your body and make you age faster. In the following chapter we will discuss what these deficiencies are—and how to avoid them.

6

How to Avoid the Deficiencies That Age You

What you habitually eat can do more than anything yet known to keep you looking and feeling younger and living longer. Or to make you age faster—and die early. "Diet is one of the most important factors in determining how long an individual lives," said Dr. Henry W. Sebrell, Jr., one of the world's leading authorities on food and its relation to a long, youthful life. "Even though you never suffer acute malnutrition," Dr. Sebrell continued, "years and years of improper eating—of dietary indiscretions—will add up to various kinds of damage to your body that will inevitably shorten your life." *The majority of men and women in their second forty years suffer from one to eight of the diseases caused by poor eating habits.*

An occasional food binge may not do any lasting harm. But if you keep on committing "dietary indiscretions" often enough —and long enough—sooner or later you'll end up with one or more of the serious deficiencies. Nutritionists and geriatricians know that diseases caused by faulty nutrition are those we can prevent, control, and in most cases reverse. But we must recognize what causes the deficiency and know what to do about it. It's easy *if you don't wait too long.*

The worst dietary indiscretions are eating too much of the

wrong foods—and not eating enough of the right ones. Most people eat too many foods high in calories, carbohydrates and fats and seem to shun the foods rich in protein, vitamins, minerals and enzymes. Overweight is one result, semistarvation and deficiency diseases are another, often at one and the same time!

It's a common mistake to assume that the fat person is well fed. *Overfed,* yes. But he is almost certain to have serious problems of malnutrition. A diet high in fats and starches, but low in the essential nutrients starves his cells, impoverishes his bloodstream, weakens his bones and muscles, raises his blood pressure, clogs his arteries, endangers his heart and shortens his life-span. Along with these harmful effects, it builds fat. So he doesn't *look* starved. And if he's young, the outward signs of his deficiencies won't show up right away. But those of us trained to observe the early symptoms of deterioration realize that before he reaches middle age he will be afflicted by some of the diseases caused by nutritional starvation. (This is not to imply that most undernourished persons are overweight—just that heavy starch eaters usually are!)

The three major deficiencies from which both fat and thin victims of malnutrition suffer are these:

1. Protein deficiency,
2. Vitamin B complex deficiency,
3. Mineral deficiency.

The way to avoid these three health wreckers that rob you of youth and vitality is to start early by making a lifetime habit of eating a variety of natural foods high in protein, vitamins and minerals.

"But I'm already middle-aged," some of you will say, "so it's too late for me to start early." Yes, it is. But you can begin *now —this very day*—to undo the damage already done. It won't be as easy as prevention, and it will take time. Remember the fellow who said, "The *difficult* is easy. The *impossible* just takes a little longer!" *From now on let every meal you eat be with a purpose—the purpose of defeating deficiencies and preventing loss of your health and youth.*

Let's take the deficiencies one at a time and see what can be done to defeat them.

Protein Deficiency

In the last chapter you learned some of the damage protein starvation can cause. For this chapter I reserved a subject of vital importance to those who, because of their religious beliefs, or for other reasons, prefer not to eat meat.

If You're a Vegetarian

Anemia is one of the problems that plague many vegetarians. Incomplete vegetable proteins *by themselves* will neither prevent nor remedy this condition. By not eating meat, especially liver, which contains iron and other blood-building factors, the vegetarian may eventually be forced to take these vital food substances in the form of injections or desiccated liver supplements.

George Bernard Shaw, a confirmed vegetarian, did this for many years. He considered concentrated liver to be his "medicine." The strict vegetarians may call this cheating, and in a way that's just what it is. It's cheating degeneration and early death, a form of cheating I heartily endorse and will help promote in every possible way!

The results of recent research in Los Angeles proved that vegetarians would be much better off if they *did* cheat. Examining the eating habits of persons between the ages of forty-five to eighty-five verified the fact that among those who ate meat there was little evidence of anemia and among non-meat eaters anemia was widely prevalent.

Persons in the over-forty age group who ate meat 1½ times a day or more (including liver once or twice a week) *had higher health scores on all counts than those who ate little or no meat.* They had more ability to resist fatigue, better reflexes, less nervousness, better condition of the eyes, of the soft tissues and of the blood. They also experienced fewer symptoms of aging deficiencies than the non-meat eaters.

An appalling number of vegetarians subsist on meals consisting mainly of protein-poor, high-starch foods. The small amount of protein they do get is not enough to protect them against illness and premature aging. The group of vegetarians who eat nuts, fruits and vegetables gets a little more protein, but still not enough!

The so-called lactovegetarians have the safest nonmeat diet. Although they prefer not to eat the biologically active meat proteins, they do allow themselves the high-grade, complete proteins of milk, milk products, eggs. But the *amount* of protein contained in these foods still falls far below that in an average serving of meat, poultry *or* fish. So the vegetarian (lacto- or otherwise) must be ever on the alert as regards protein intake.

This means that even the lactovegetarian must eat larger amounts of food than the meat eater if he is to keep his protein intake high enough to avoid deficiencies. Unless they fortify their nutritionally inadequate meals with enough of the complete, concentrated vegetable proteins to prevent it, the "hidden hunger" of vegetarians often causes them to gorge on carbohydrates. And that can be a serious threat to health and life.

BEST VEGETABLE PROTEINS

Group I

(complete and highly concentrated)

Food	*Amount*	*Approx. Protein Grams*
Brewer's yeast	½ cup	40
Millet meal	1 cup	34
Sesame seed meal	1 cup	27
Soybean flour	1 cup	40
Soybeans, dried	1 cup	20
Soybeans, fresh	1 cup	16
Sunflower seed meal	1 cup	40
Wheat germ	½ cup	24

Group II

(incomplete, but good quality and quantity)

Food	*Amount*	*Approx. Protein Grams*
Barley, whole	1 cup	16
Cornmeal, unbolted	1 cup	12
Kidney beans	½ cup	6
Lentils	½ cup	9
Lima beans, dried	½ cup	8
Lima beans, green	½ cup	7
Peanut butter	4 tbsp.	18
Peanut flour	1 cup	59
Peas, dried	½ cup	12
Peas, fresh	½ cup	7
Parsley	½ cup	6
Whole wheat flour	1 cup	12

Group III

(Nuts are listed in a separate group, because, although they contain a good grade of protein, with two exceptions, it's in surprisingly small amounts.)

Food	*Amount*	*Approx. Protein Grams*
Almonds	½ cup	13.2
Cashews	15	3
Chestnuts	18	3
Peanuts	½ cup	19
Pecans	15	3
Walnuts	15	2

If you're a vegetarian, do make liberal use of some or all of the concentrated complete vegetable proteins as often as you can. Since soybeans are a superior source of all the essential amino acids they should be staples of your diet.

When you eat macaroni and spaghetti (though not too often), get the kind made with protein-rich soy flour. For added flavor and enrichment, sprinkle meatless dishes generously with sunflower seeds, sesame seeds or wheat germ. Top salads with the same high-protein seeds or with wheat germ. Add sunflower seed meal to cooked cereal. Try millet as a cooked cereal or as a nutritious substitute for potatoes or rice.

You *can* avoid deficiencies on a vegetarian diet if you supplement it with concentrated vegetable proteins and don't limit yourself to foods containing little or no protein. *And remember that the need for protein increases rather than decreases with the years.*

Most of the complete protein foods also contain an abundance of B vitamins. If you're protein-starved, you may well be a victim of some of the physical, mental and emotional ills brought on by a vitamin B complex shortage. And that leads us into the second major deficiency!

B Complex Deficiency

The following list of symptoms and diseases all have one thing in common: They can be caused by a deficiency ranging from mild to acute of one or more of the B vitamins:

Chronic exhaustion
Craving for sweets and/or alcohol
Loss of appetite and weight
Digestive disturbances
Extreme nervousness
Insomnia
Dermatitis and other skin diseases
Degeneration of nerve cells
Loss of courage and ambition
Mental confusion and severe depression
Hostility, suspicion and other paranoid symptoms
Juvenile delinquency

And these are only a *few* of the conditions that can result from this second major deficiency! Of course, serious conditions should be treated professionally. To avoid deficiencies and to correct those not requiring therapeutic measures, let B-rich foods be your medicine. Add B complex supplements when necessary.

All of the complete animal protein foods listed in the previous chapter are good sources of B vitamins: meat, poultry, fish, powdered skim milk and buttermilk. Yogurt is especially desirable, because it manufactures B vitamins in your own intestinal tract.

Leafy greens, eaten raw or very lightly cooked, contain moderate amounts, and avocado is an excellent source of B_1, a good source of niacin, and a fair source of B_2 (all members of the B complex family). Liver and brewer's yeast are probably the two richest sources of B complex vitamins. Wheat germ is the third best source. Of special interest to women is that B complex vitamins are beneficial to the skin, helping to keep it smooth, unblemished, youthful.

Mineral Deficiency

A staggering ninety-nine percent of our population suffers to some extent from mineral deficiency. If you are one of them, the chances are you're also suffering in varying degrees from all three deficiencies!

Lacking the dramatic appeal of vitamins, minerals have become the Cinderella of the food element family. This is unfortunate indeed, since minerals—just as vitamins and proteins—are vitally essential regulators and builders of the billions of living cell units which make up the human body.

When your group of cells becomes ill-fed and only half-alive, you may say that you feel "sluggish, dopey." What you are actually admitting is that your body is starved.

Government researchers reported that "a marked deficiency in any one of the more important minerals results in disease."

The document continues, repeating the dangers I've warned of for years (and sometimes been called an alarmist for it!), "*Any upset of the balance, any considerable lack of one or another element, however microscopic the body requirement may be, and we sicken, suffer, shorten our lives.*" (My italics)

The average adult is generally more deficient in calcium than in any other single mineral. This is a serious deficiency since every muscle in your body—including your heart muscle—needs calcium for strength and muscle tone. Muscle tissues irritated by a calcium shortage are a major cause of foot and leg cramps. And without calcium to aid blood clotting, an injured person can bleed to death.

To keep bones and teeth strong as you grow older, an abundance of both vitamin D and calcium are necessary. When bones or teeth are poorly calcified, they degenerate and crumble or break easily. A slight stumble or minor twist can cause the fractures and breaks that occur often in older persons whose demineralized bones have become as fragile and porous as honeycomb. Called *osteoporosis,* this condition responds favorably, even in advanced cases, to calcium and vitamin D. But how much better to avoid the deficiency that causes it!

Calcium also aids the transmittal of nerve impulses. A deficiency may first show up in tense nerves, irritability, temper flare-ups, fatigue, inability to relax, insomnia. When adequate calcium is supplied and reaches the nerves, these symptoms are soon relieved. But the cup of warm milk at bedtime, often recommended to calm nerves and relieve insomnia, doesn't supply enough calcium to benefit the person who is seriously deficient and who may fail to absorb it.

One problem in the body's utilization of calcium is that there are many factors that inhibit its absorption. One of them is the decrease of hydrochloric acid in the stomach as we grow older. Without it, calcium remains insoluble and can't be assimilated. Yogurt and buttermilk are far superior to the other calcium-rich milk products, because of their lactic acid content that substitutes for hydrochloric acid and makes the calcium usable.

A high-protein diet aids calcium retention. So do vitamin D and the unsaturated fatty acids (preferably safflower oil). However, solid, saturated fats, white sugar, cocoa and chocolate inhibit calcium absorption. Instead of cocoa, stir a tablespoon of blackstrap molasses in a cup of milk, and you'll get an additional 116 milligrams of calcium, a hefty helping of iron and some of the B complex—all in one spoonful!

BEST FOOD SOURCES OF CALCIUM

Almonds	Dates
Apricots, dried	Figs, fresh and dried
Avocado	Leafy green vegetables, all kinds
Bananas	Powdered skim milk
Bean sprouts	Soy flour
Blackstrap molasses	Soybeans, dried
Brewer's yeast	Wheat germ
Buttermilk	Whole wheat
Cheese, all unprocessed	Yogurt
Clams	

For years I've been telling my students that "life of the flesh is in the blood." A healthy bloodstream is your lifestream. It carries oxygen and sustenance to your cells and renewed vitality to all parts of your body. It gives your skin its glow and your lips and cheeks their youthful color.

But it can do all of these things only if the red blood cells contain their full quota of hemoglobin. Without this essential "coloring content" of the red blood cells, they become as pale and washed-out as the anemic person suffering from low hemoglobin and what television commercials call "tired blood." You've heard announcers describe the dragging symptoms caused by iron-poor blood—and for once they aren't exaggerating!

Where I disagree with them is in the remedy. The red blood cells themselves are made of protein, and hemoglobin consists largely of protein and iron. Certain of the B vitamins also contribute to their health. A serious lack of any essential food element sets the stage for the appearance of other deficiencies. When red blood cells are starved of protein, B vitamins and the minerals iron, copper and iodine, the inevitable result is "tired blood," iron-deficiency anemia—or worse.

The Food and Nutrition Board of the National Research Council recommends twelve milligrams of iron a day for adults (fifteen for adolescents and pregnant or lactating women), but this is a bare minimum. Better double the amount to be safe, and raise it 100 percent if a deficiency already exists. And remember that women need more iron than men. You don't have to count milligrams to be sure of getting enough. Just eat a variety of the foods listed as your best sources of protein and B vitamins, especially the following:

BEST FOOD SOURCES OF IRON

- Apricots
- Barley, whole
- Beef heart
- Beef tongue
- Beet greens
- Clams
- Dates
- Egg yolks
- Kidney
- Kidney and lima beans
- Liver, all kinds
- Molasses, blackstrap
- Mustard greens
- Parsley
- Peanut flour
- Peanuts
- Soybean sprouts
- Soybeans, dried
- Soybean flour
- Sunflower seeds
- Swiss chard
- Wheat germ
- Whole wheat flour

All meats contain considerable amounts of iron, but I omitted muscle meats in favor of organ meats on this list, because a larger percentage of their iron content is assimilated.

To prevent iron-poor blood, depend on these foods and enough physical activity to stimulate circulation—*never* on any patent medicine, whether it's spelled backward, forward, or sideways. And be sure you're not deficient in hydrochloric acid, which dissolves the iron and aids its assimilation by the body. But don't take any chances with pernicious anemia. Get professional help for that.

While many minerals are liberally supplied in a variety of everyday foods, iodine is not. Yet if you're deficient in this one mineral, it can affect not only your hemoglobin sufficiency, but your energy, nerves, weight, skin, hair and entire appearance. It takes only a slight trace of iodine to make the difference between quick perception and sluggish apathy, between the mental giant and the plodding dullard.

You won't risk a deficiency of iodine if you include plenty of ocean fish in your diet. Also now recognized as an important iodine food are Massachusetts cranberries or other cranberries grown in similar soil near the sea.

But the highest concentration of iodine (and almost all the other minerals) is found in the dried-sea-vegetation products available in health food stores: dulse, kelp, sea lettuce and Irish moss. Try the dehydrated flakes in soups, stews, and as seasoning. (Kelp is available in tablet form, too.) The least they can do is boost your iodine intake, your energy and—who knows?—maybe your intelligence. Whether you need it or not!

In addition to calcium, iron and iodine, the body requires many other minerals even though only in *microscopic* quantities. But without that small fraction, that "trace" of these minerals, we "sicken, suffer, shorten our lives."

A basic knowledge of minerals and the part they play in maintaining body health is an important step toward a good understanding of nutrition as applied to everyday living.

Dr. W. C. Rose, professor of nutrition at the University of Illinois, says: "The chemical elements which make up the body sustenance must be nicely balanced or trouble ensues. The efficiency of each element is enhanced by proper amounts of the others."

Biochemistry has proved over and over again that our health can be no better than our mineral balance. That is why I urge you to pay more attention to minerals in your diet; otherwise you may suffer needlessly from mental upsets and physical ailments that have their only basis in mineral starvation of the body's cells.

Because it is not always possible to so balance meals that all the essential minerals will be included in the diet every day, the prudent person will, in addition to carefully planned meals, also use a reliable mineral food supplement each day as "dietary insurance."

It's up to you to avoid or remedy all deficiencies with a diet rich in protein, vitamins and minerals, plus the concentrated foods and supplements recommended for specific deficiencies. Correct the deficiencies, avoid the disabling diseases they cause, help your cells renew themselves and you can, as Dr. Tom Spies said, "make old age wait"—far longer than you ever believed possible!

One disease that is believed to be induced or accelerated by nutrient deficiencies is cancer. Much research must still be done before we have any definitive answers about the nature and best means of prevention and cure for this dreaded killer. But in the next chapter we will see what science has discovered about the relationship between diet and cancer.

7

Cancer—a Deficiency Disease?

Cancer claims over 300,000 lives a year. Yet there are several ways of protecting yourself and your family from this formidable killer—*if you start in time*. My purpose is to help you build up all the protection you can against the disease and to tell you of ways that have been effective in decreasing susceptibility to it. I want to establish at the outset that I will not hold out to anyone the false hope of a cure until there is positive proof that one has been discovered.

Cancer research is still going on and great progress is being made. There is real hope that an eventual cure will be found, though how it will happen and how long it will take are not yet known. Hope carries with it no guarantee of how or when. Instead, let's see what the very real hope of *prevention* can offer.

At Auburn University in Alabama a four-man research team headed by Dr. W. D. Salmon recently combined for the first time the factors of nutrition, biochemistry and pathology in simultaneous laboratory studies of diet deficiencies in white rats, chickens and dogs. These specialists in four different fields arrived at the same conclusion: *A diet deficient in certain essential nutrients causes cancer in animals!* But what about human beings? Do the same deficiencies make *them* susceptible to cancer?

In the conservative way of researchers, Dr. Salmon answered this question by saying, "If we knew that these things occurred only in animals, we wouldn't be much interested in continuing."

Their experiments have not been limited to cancer research alone. They also found that when animals were fed a high-fat diet deficient in the B vitamin element choline, these animals suffered the same degeneration of heart muscles and blood vessels that we already know occurs in man on the same diet.

What may have an important bearing on cancer prevention in man is their discovery that a deficiency of *only one B vitamin* (choline) caused the test animals to develop cancer "within an astonishingly short time."

Other experiments showing the effectiveness of B vitamins in cancer prevention were conducted some years ago by Dr. Kanematsu Sugiura at the Sloan-Kettering Institute for Cancer Research in New York City. Dr. Sugiura produced liver cancer in rats in 150 days by keeping them on a vitamin-deficient diet of polished rice and a cancer-inducing substance called butter yellow (once used to color margarine but now prohibited). Next, he fed four new groups of rats the same cancer-causing diet, but in addition, three of the groups received daily amounts of brewer's yeast in the respective proportions of three percent, six percent and fifteen percent.

Within 150 days, all the rats in the group that received no brewer's yeast were as positive as Dr. Sugiura's. He also discovered that desiccated liver, containing a high concentration of amount of brewer's yeast in the diet increased, the incidence of cancer decreased. Less than a third of those receiving six percent contracted the disease. And of the animals that were given the most yeast, fifteen percent, not one showed any sign of cancer!

A follow-up of these experiments was made by a pioneer researcher, Dr. Boris Sokoloff. His results with the vitamin B-rich brewer's yeast were as positive as Dr. Sugiura's. He also discovered that desiccated liver, containing a high concentration of B vitamins, had a cancer preventive effect equal to that of yeast. In an article in the *Journal of Nutrition* Dr. Sugiura concluded: "These dietary influences [brewer's yeast and desiccated liver] may prove to play a very large part in the causation, prevention and treatment of human cancer."

But time went by and countless lives were lost before "dietary influences and their relation to cancer" were regarded as more than theories—except, of course, by nutritionists. It isn't enough to have experiments that offer proof in animals and hope for humans if the results are unheard by those who would benefit by them and ignored by those who hear. Strong voices of authority are needed to make the facts now available concerning cancer prevention heard and believed.

Here are the voices of some leading authorities now speaking out on the subject.

In Lindau, Germany, in July, 1966, at a meeting of the Nobel Prize winners for that year, Dr. Otto Warburg, director of the Max Planck Institute for Cell Physiology in Berlin, gave an address "Concerning the Ultimate Cause and the Contributing Causes of Cancer." He took into consideration the many known cancer-inducers, including radiation, harmful chemicals, deficiencies, and a weakness or error in the metabolism. He then reduced them all to one primary cause: the lack of one or more of three B vitamins—riboflavin, niacin and pantothenic acid—in the tissues where the tumor forms.

Dr. Warburg heralded these three vitamins as the substances that would give human beings the best possible chance of avoiding cancer. Not animals, as American experiments had already proved, *but human beings!* His confidence in the power of these vitamins to arrest malignant growths was so strong that he advised their use to prevent the spread of cancer or its recurrence following surgery.

Dr. Warburg explained it this way: The oxidation of food for the cells' use requires oxygen. A thirty-five percent reduction of the oxygen available to the cell causes it to switch to another metabolic process in its fight to survive, and it gets its sustenance instead from fermenting sugar.

Almost twenty years ago, in one of my books, *Health Through Nutrition,* I wrote of the link between cancer and the overconsumption of sugar and starch, and described how the abnormal cells compete with healthy ones for the nourishment that means their survival. Here is what I said at that time:

> . . . Whatever nourishment is present will be taken up at once by the normal cells, leaving the cancerous cells to thrive as best they can on whatever food surplus there may be . . . But, *if there is a superabundance of body sugars in the tissue fluid, derived from carbohydrate foods in the diet, then the cancerous cells will have found the nourishment to make them grow and thrive, and the abnormal growth progresses to its third and final stage.*

Recently a Nobel Prize winner of the University of Pennsylvania Medical School, Dr. Otto Meyerhoff, spoke of the evidence connecting the excessive consumption of sugar with cancer by calling attention to "the appetite of tumors for sugar." He suggested that the growth of cancerous tissue might possibly be stopped if biochemists could find a way of curing this appetite.

A high-protein diet and B vitamins have been given credit as aids to cancer prevention by many American researchers. The hope that Dr. Sugiura had of protecting humans from cancer with brewer's yeast is proving to be a viable method. The same amount of yeast that gave full protection to test animals long ago has now been recommended for humans by Dr. H. F. Kraybill of the National Cancer Research.

In *Clinical Pharmacology and Therapeutics* Dr. Kraybill wrote:

> Yeast [rich in B vitamins] is particularly effective for the prevention of liver cancer since the level of 15 percent of it is almost completely protective, and *any high-quality protein diet and B vitamins, especially B-2* [*riboflavin*], *are defensive mechanisms in inhibiting the formations of such neoplasms* [*abnormal growths or cancer*]. (My italics and parenthetical notes)

Cancer and Deficiency

The identification of protein and B vitamins as the body's defense mechanisms that inhibit the growth of tumors is in line with the belief of other prominent researchers that cancer is a deficiency disease.

Dr. J. R. Davidson, a former associate professor of clinical medicine at the University of Manitoba, stated: "I believe cancer, a deficiency disease, can be prevented and controlled by a suitable and balanced diet, high in vitamin content." Dr. Davidson stressed the fact that such a diet would act to *prevent* cancer, not cure it. Yet in many of the patients he treated who "suffered from clearly diagnosed cancers of severe degree," some improvement occurred.

The diet prescribed by Dr. Davidson, while varying to some extent in each individual case, includes one pint of freshly made vegetable juice per day (such as carrot, lettuce and celery juices), plenty of raw vegetables (particularly peas, beans, carrots, spinach, lettuce), wheat germ (another good source of B vitamins), meat cooked rare, raw milk, and concentrated vitamins of various kinds.

An Omaha, Nebraska, cancer specialist, D. T. Quigley, M.D., had no recurrence of cancer in hundreds of patients who followed his prescribed diet, which is similar to Dr. Davidson's. Dr. Quigley's successful treatment was based on the premise that cancer "never grows on healthy tissues, but always on previously diseased tissues." In his diet, to keep the cells and tissues healthy and to build up the body's resistance to cancer, Dr. Quigley *absolutely prohibited all refined, synthetic and processed food, including white flour, white sugar and all products with chemical additives.*

These are the foods that prevented a recurrence of cancer in the patients he treated: Liberal amounts of protein (meat, fish, poultry and eggs), whole grains and all natural, whole foods, raw vegetables and fruits and raw certified milk, *plus all the known natural vitamins and minerals, including the finest natural sources of B vitamins, brewer's yeast, liver and wheat germ.*

That the healthy body does build up its own immunity against cancer was first proved in tests with volunteer prisoners at Ohio State Penitentiary and with patients at Memorial Hospital, New York City. When cancer cells were injected into *healthy* tissues, the results were only the soreness and minor discomforts of an ordinary vaccination. But in cases where cancer cells were injected into *diseased* tissues, cancer developed. As Dr. Cornelius P. Rhoads, of the Sloan-Kettering Institute, reported, "The healthy ones threw off cancer as easily as they did a common cold, whereas others were easy victims of it."

The results of other successful experiments in the nutritional approach to cancer, conducted under the supervision of Dr. Robert D. Barnard, consultant to the Cancer Research Division of the Department of Health, New York City, were published in the New York *Times*, September 3, 1960. Here is the conclusion of that report:

". . . Cancer is merely a local manifestation of a body-wide deficiency and can sometimes be treated by feeding patients substances that accelerate cell growth."

The fact that Dr. Barnard's report was read to the Fifth International Congress on *Nutrition* before it was published suggests that nutritional methods may be effective not merely in the prevention of cancer, but in the *treatment* of cancer.

Whether or not scientists are prepared to name the specific nutritional deficiencies that result in cancer (as a few have done), the majority of them agree on the two principal factors involved: some form of deficiency and some form of irritation. Alexander Berglas, member of the Cancer Research Foundation of the Pasteur Institute, Paris, France, summed it up in one sentence: *"Irritation and deficiency factors will cause the regulatory mechanism (of the body) to fail."* (My italics)

Some known and suspected contributing causes are vitamin B deficiency, a hormone imbalance, viral infections, chronic infections that cause constant irritation, ultraviolet ray, x-ray, radium, atomic fission, trauma (from injuries, accidents or operations). Among the many chemical irritants are the dangerous coal tar and nicotine in cigarettes.

In the chapter on habits, I report recent experiments that showed the value of vitamins C and A in protecting the smoker from lung cancer. According to the *Journal of the American Medical Association* (8:14:54), two German doctors have for some years successfully treated cancer in other areas of the body with 1,000 milligrams of vitamin C and massive doses of vitamin A each day. (I am purposely omitting the amount of vitamin A used, since such a high intake of it is not advised except under the strictest supervision.) Under this treatment, the natural defenses of the cells improved, healing occurred in cancerous ulcers of the cervix and rectum, the general condition of all the patients improved, and even in advanced cases where the tumors were not healed, there was a significant decrease in size.

From *Nutrition Abstracts and Reviews* comes a later report from Germany on this treatment, which is now being administered by injection for fourteen to twenty-one days, vitamin C intravenously and vitamin A intramuscularly. After that, large amounts are given by mouth, as in the earlier treatment. In all patients treated, according to the recent report, "The effect was generally good and growth of the tumor became stationary or regressed. The treatment should be regarded as auxiliary, not as in itself curative. No side effects of excess of vitamins were seen."

Making the nutritional means of protection a part of your overall preventive plan can do no less than improve your health —and the evidence gives hope that some of them could save your life. The American Society for Microbiology says this about cancer prevention:

> . . . Cancer cells arise constantly in the body but are usually killed by defense mechanisms . . . Reinforcement in a general way of the body's natural defenses . . . might prevent the development of malignancies. (Reported by John A. Osmundsen in the New York *Times,* May 7, 1964)

Here are more of the general ways that have proved helpful in reinforcing those defenses.

From *Medical World News* comes recent information concerning the apparent anticancerous effect of yogurt and kefir:

> The harmless rod-shaped organism which makes yogurt out of milk (and kefir), Lactobacillus bulgaricus, turns out to have a

> potent antitumor activity, according to researchers at the Bulgarian Academy of Sciences in Solla. Injections of Lactobacillus bulgaricus extracts, they say, can cure several types of experimental cancers and appear to be effective against human skin tumors.

The report continues by quoting Dr. Ivan Bogdanov, of the academy's Scientific Research Institute for Anticancer Antibodies: "Hundreds of mice have been 'completely cured' of usually lethal advanced sarcomas and ascites tumors. Moreover, animals thus cured are immune to further transplants of the same tumor . . ."

The lactic acid treatment of a European researcher, Dr. Johannes Kuhl, has much in common with the Bulgarian experiments, since yogurt, kefir and buttermilk are all rich in lactic acid. After more than 1,000 successful experiments, Dr. Kuhl concluded that these two factors offer protection against cancer:

1. Reinforcing a wholesome, natural diet of the essential nutrients with liberal daily amounts of the lactic-acid fermented foods. (Among them are yogurt, kefir, buttermilk, clabber or other soured milk, cottage cheese, and such lactic-acid fermented vegetables as sauerkraut, pickled beets and pickled cucumbers.)
2. Eliminating or reducing to an absolute minimum sweets, and *all* processed, devitalized foods, including white sugar, white flour and other high-carbohydrate products.

In Tokyo, at the Ninth International Cancer Congress in 1966 (where Dr. Saffiotti reported the prevention of lung cancer with vitamin A), Japanese scientists told of their extensive series of experiments that showed how milk inhibits or prevents the development of stomach cancer.

It's been more than thirty years since it was proved that calcium inhibits the growth of certain cancers in mice. By adding calcium lactate to the diet of mice, Drs. Max Goldzieher, E. Rosenthal and Z. Mizuna produced amazing results: *The mouse cancers calcified, and their growth was stopped.*

One of the world's leading authorities on the bacteriological approach to cancer reports on a little-known deficiency, that of an enzyme, *catalase,* and its relation to the disease. He is R. A. Holman, M.D., honorary consultant bacteriologist, United Cardiff Hospitals, and senior lecturer, School of Medicine, University of Wales. Here are excerpts from his famous treatise on the contributing causes of cancer and what can be done about them:

> As a result of the rapid technological advances, large numbers of physical and chemical agents have been placed or released into man's external and internal environment with little thought about the possible long-term effect of these on his own cells . . . The real attack on the treatment of malignant growths must come from intelligent interference with the catalase-peroxide mechanism [catalase is a body enzyme] . . .
>
> To develop a far more effective cure it is essential that the catalase-peroxide mechanism be exploited in order to determine the most efficient way of over-oxidizing the catalase-deficient cells . . .
>
> The plan for prevention of cancer should be threefold:
>
> 1. To increase our intake of catalase.
>
> Catalase, as well as many other enzymes, is destroyed by heat. Civilized man now lives primarily out of the can, the bottle and the package . . . *It would be to everyone's advantage if the consumption of fresh fruits and vegetables were to be markedly increased, thus ensuring a far greater intake of catalase and peroxidase.* [My italics] There are numerous references in the literature to the fact that garlic-eating people have an increased resistance to cancer. This is not surprising when one realizes that garlic is very rich in the catalytic systems containing catalase and peroxidase.
>
> 2. To increase the manufacture of catalase by our own cells.
>
> . . . If a normally active creature is forcibly imprisoned in a cage so as to limit its normal activity, then after some weeks the catalase content of the body decreases. Conversely, normally inactive creatures can be made to develop more catalase if forcibly exercised. It is very probable, therefore, that the chronic habit of limiting the muscular activity of man . . . in cars, trains and other forms of mechanical locomotion . . . is doing much to diminish his normal catalase level . . . In general, a higher concentration

of catalase implies an increased consumption of oxygen which provides a catalytic system of prime importance in the detoxification of our bodies.

3. To curtail the intake of agents which destroy or inhibit the action of our cell catalase.

. . . It has been estimated that there are now more than 1,000 additives to our food and drink. Many of these interfere with the catalase-peroxide balance.

Chemical agents have been added to food and drink . . . to kill bacteria, resulting in a longer shelf life; to color the products . . . to act as sweeteners, flavoring agents, etc.; to accelerate the growth of chickens, bullocks, fish, etc. . . .

. . . The control of air pollution demands our most urgent attention. A good oxygen intake is essential . . . for the removal and destruction of many toxic agents present in or on our cells . . .

Many drugs now used can interfere with cell respiration . . .

X-rays and other forms of irradiation are known to inhibit catalase . . .

Cancer prevention, the only effective, scientific method of controlling the disease, can show results if we pull together and reform some of our bad habits so prevalent in our civilized way of living.

(For more on enzymes, see Chapter 10.)

Avoid These Cancer Inducers:

Don't eat *any* kind of dyed food. That includes colored nuts, desserts and bakery foods, dyed oranges and potatoes, margarine colored with anything except carotene (a natural color).

Throw away the necks of chicken and turkey (that's where the chemicals are injected), and never eat capon at all.

Remove burned edges and charred fats from overcooked meats and poultry. Throw away burned toast instead of scraping it. Carefully trim all burned, charred or tarry substances from food. And don't ever order a steak "rare in the middle and burned on the outside"!

Don't get fat. If you're already overweight, reduce to normal. Cancer is more likely to strike the overweight than the slender.

Don't overeat. Cut down on foods that are high in calories, carbohydrates and fats. But eat plenty of high-grade proteins and vitamin-and-mineral-rich vegetables and fruits, as many raw as you can.

Avoid white sugar, white flour and all processed, refined foods. Use pepper and spices in moderation.

Don't gulp down scalding cups of soup, coffee or other hot beverage. They'll taste just as good—or better—if they don't burn all the way down.

Avoid any known or suspected type of deficiency. If your food doesn't supply the necessary nutrients or if your absorption is poor, supplement your diet with concentrated food products. Use a good B complex *and* a complete, well-balanced multivitamin-mineral supplement.

There are many types of cancer and many methods of treatment. But the recommendations for protection against all the various types of cancer have three common purposes: to correct nutritional deficiencies, to avoid chemical imbalances, and to build up the body's defenses against the disease in whatever way is indicated. By building up your body and strengthening its natural defenses in the methods recommended for protection, you will, as Dr. Warburg said, *"give yourself the best possible chance of avoiding cancer."*

Correcting deficiencies is, however, only one part of a two-pronged attack on health problems related to nutrition. The other essential is to avoid the foods that actually rob the body of necessary nutrients and thereby promote physical decline and rapid aging.

8

Beware of Foods That Can Be Killers!

Are you a sugar addict? "Well, I like desserts and candy," many of you will admit and then go on to protest, "but I'm not *addicted* to anything." I don't like the word "addict" either. But it sounds a little nicer than another word I could use for it —sugar *drunk*.

Sugar and starch addiction can fasten itself upon men, women or children. It has a special affinity for those who are unable to relate or communicate successfully with others: the failures, the disappointed and frustrated, the emotionally unstable and insecure.

Such persons find comfort and a temporary escape in sweets and high-starch foods that turn to sugar when digested. In a way this is comparable to the alcoholic who turns to liquor rather than face his problems. Just as there are compulsive, solitary drinkers, so are there compulsive, solitary carbohydrate addicts. Like the alcoholic who hides his bottle and drinks in secret, many confirmed sugar addicts hide their chocolates, cookies, and other sweets. Gobbling them up becomes a private affair. Here's how Dr. Edward Weiss, writing in *Journal of Clinical Nutrition,* describes compulsive sugar and starch eaters: ". . . The eating is like an obsession—*indeed, very much like addiction to alcohol.*" (My italics)

Alcoholics Anonymous bases its treatment of alcoholism on the knowledge that in extreme cases *there is no tapering off*. The patient must be prevented from taking that one drink that will topple him off the wagon. The same is true of sugar addicts. One taste of anything sweet is their downfall. They are absolutely incapable of eating just *one* piece of candy, one cookie or small slice of cake or pie.

One bite of any dessert will do to satisfy the normal person's occasional craving for forbidden foods. But sugar addicts are not normal. They may, for example, be victims of low blood sugar.

Other compulsive eaters are food neurotics who have regressed to a childhood pattern. They associate candy, ice cream, pudding, other sweets and soft, starchy foods with the "reward" foods their mothers gave them when they were good. They grow up and find that the world doesn't reward and appreciate them as their parents did. So they "reward" themselves—by continually gorging on the foods that once made them happy. The approach to their problem is a little different.

Ava Bennet, a food neurotic who once consulted me, was suffering from an insatiable hunger for the high-carbohydrate foods that were responsible for her low blood sugar. And her low blood sugar was responsible for her loss of energy and ambition, severe mental and emotional disturbances and the wreck of her looks and once charming, dynamic personality. Her husband had left her, and her physical and emotional strength was ebbing.

When she opened the door to greet me, she burst into hysterical weeping. I led her to a chair and went to the kitchen to get her a glass of water. A box of sugar-coated cereal was on the drainboard, and one sweet roll remained in a package that had contained six.

I began to see the extent to which she had come to depend on sweet foods and drinks when I opened her refrigerator—and all but shuddered at its contents! Rows of sweetened, carbonated drinks lined the shelves. A huge pizza stood in the center, surrounded by half a Dutch chocolate cake, three chocolate eclairs, the remains of a butterscotch pie and a box of chocolates.

I opened the freezer compartment and saw large cartons of ice cream and frozen chocolate-coated pies. I shuddered at the horrifying thought that a human being was killing herself by trying to exist on the contents of this kitchen—foods loaded with sugar, starch and fats, absolutely deficient in protein, vitamins and minerals!

When I returned, Ava told me why her husband had left her. "Look at me," she said despairingly. "Can you blame him?" I looked at the deep lines and bags under the red-rimmed eyes, the blotchy skin, the heavy jowls and folds of flesh that hid the fine bone structure of her face and body, the swollen hands and legs.

"What happened to you?" I asked.

"That's just what I was going to ask you," she said. "What's wrong with me? Can you help me?"

"Yes, I can," I said, "but you'll have to cooperate. When your husband was away, were you hungry all the time, especially for sweets and starches?"

"I gobbled them constantly," she replied. "I hated myself for it. But I felt so sorry for myself and so frustrated and miserable that I couldn't stop eating. Each time Ward returned from a sales trip I looked more repulsive. I knew I was unbearably nervous and irritable, but I couldn't help it, even when I saw he could hardly wait to get away from me again."

"Didn't you try to do anything about it?" I asked.

"I didn't know what to do. I felt lost and confused. There were times I thought I was losing my mind. Eating was the only comfort I had. So I kept right on stuffing myself."

"Why didn't you go back to work, volunteer for some community service or go out with friends?" I asked. "Anything that would keep you occupied and keep your mind off your troubles —and food."

"I'm ashamed to have anyone see me. And I couldn't type—look at my hands!" She held out her stiff and swollen fingers. "Besides, half the time I'm so dizzy I have to lie down, or I'd black out. And most of the time I'm in such a state of mental confusion I can't think straight. Right now I feel ready to faint —if I don't have some food this very minute!" I didn't try to stop her as she got unsteadily to her feet and waddled—there's no other word for it—toward the kitchen.

After she had wolfed down a large dish of ice cream she admitted, "I have to eat so often—and so much. I can't help it. I get weak, confused and dizzy and feel absolutely starved if I don't."

"Of course, you do," I said. "You *are* absolutely starved. You're inviting physical and mental degeneration—and death! —by depriving yourself of essential nutrients. The junk you've been eating is incapable of sustaining life. Sugar gives you a momentary lift by raising your blood sugar level—then almost immediately plunges it down to rock bottom again, making you feel worse than ever. You create a vicious cycle by eating more and more sugar, which increases the erratic rise and fall of blood sugar, and starves your brain of glucose and your body of its nerve-stabilizing B vitamins and other nutrients. It *increases* your craving for sweets and leads to a whole series of deficiencies that affect your body, mind and nervous system."

"What started this chain reaction?" Ava asked. "I used to be a healthy person with a normal appetite—except that sometimes I'd crave something sweet when I'd get nervous and upset."

She admitted to having been upset most of the time since she and her husband started having trouble.

I explained to her the relationship between psychological state and the sugar levels of the body: "Emotional upsets overstimulate the sensitive pancreas, causing it to produce too much insulin. The function of insulin is to neutralize excess sugar. This causes a sharp drop in the blood sugar level. Too much insulin and the resulting low blood sugar are responsible for many hard-to-diagose ills. Among its many symptoms are those you have—confusion, dizziness, irritability, exhaustion, an inordinate craving for sweets—and worse."

In an address to an American Medical Association meeting in New York, Dr. Stephen P. Gyland, Sr., said this about the functional type of low blood sugar, or hyperinsulinism, known as hypoglycemia: "There is probably no illness today which . . . causes such widespread suffering as that of hypoglycemia. So much inefficiency and loss of time. So many accidents. So many family breakups. And so many suicides."

The Hypoglycemia Foundation applauded Dr. Gyland's address but added that he might have gone on to point out that in most cases controlling low blood sugar is relatively simple. (It's the diagnosis that's difficult, since it sneaks up on you, wearing as many disguises as the villain in an old silent movie.) "Such control," the Foundati[illegible]ould often go a long way in preventing diabetes an[illegible]enia, reducing alcoholism, juvenile delinquency, r[illegible]s, chronic fatigue, asthma, allergies, and so many [illegible] and common social problems."

"Isn't it logical to e[illegible] sweet to raise the blood sugar?" asked Ava.

"That mistake is often [illegible] "But it's the worst thing you can do—except as a [illegible] measure. Only protein foods will keep the blood [illegible]ven level and avoid the drastic rises and sudden d[illegible]ges caused by sugar."

In the majority of cases, [illegible] sugar and other high carbohydrates, which the dig[illegible]s turns into sugar, are responsible for low blood suga[illegible]od sugar can also be caused by drugs and stimulants, i[illegible]alcohol, which is both a stimulant and a carbohydrate. Stre[illegible]ch as anxiety, worry, fear and grief trigger the condition b[illegible]epleting the adrenal cortical reserves. This overstimulates the pancreas so it produces excessive amounts of insulin, which burn up the blood sugar.

"Because of their dangerously high sugar and starch diets," I said, "millions are suffering from low blood sugar—or its direct opposite, diabetes."

"You say they're direct opposites?" Ava asked. "Then how is it possible for the same diet to cause both?"

"Let's break it down into three conditions of the pancreas," I said. "The island of Langerhans in the pancreas secretes insulin, which neutralizes sugar and keeps an excess of it from suddenly pouring into the circulation.

"The normal pancreas secretes the exact amount of insulin needed to keep the blood sugar level under control. (But don't overload it with sugar, starch and fats, or it won't stay normal!)

"Next is the pancreas that produces *too little insulin to neutralize the sugar,* causing a drastic rise in blood sugar that results in diabetes, which can be a killer. To stay alive, the diabetic must remain on a controlled diet that eliminates sugar. He may, in addition, require injections of insulin.

"The pancreas that secretes *too much insulin* has just the opposite effect. The excess of insulin neutralizes too much sugar, which consequently results in *low blood sugar,* often called the sugar disease, but known medically as hyperinsulinism, or hypoglycemia."

If you suffer from low blood sugar, you may feel as Ava did when she asked, "What do you think is wrong with me—besides *everything?*" Everything, it seems, *is* wrong with you. If you're nervous and high-strung to begin with, you grow worse as your own tensions consume your blood sugar. Tension mounts as you fight the severe headaches, the rigid, muscle-bound neck and shoulders, the stiff and aching joints, the stomach pains, the attacks of heart palpitation, the dizziness and the inability to concentrate or make a decision. Depression and anxieties engulf you. Disposition drops from good to bad to terrible.

As confusion and mental apathy close in upon you, you wonder, as Ava did, if you're losing your mind. How else could you feel since your brain cells are the first to starve? The brain can't store sugar for future use, as other organs can. For its sustenance, it must have glucose from moment to moment. It's absolutely impossible to think clearly, work efficiently and live normally when your blood sugar level is too low to supply the needs of your brain, nerve and muscle cells.

But let me repeat this maxim so you'll always remember it: *Eating sugar is not the remedy. Protein foods are the only ones that can keep your blood sugar at a normal level and prevent the erratic rises and downward plunges that carbohydrates cause it to take! Sugar in any form is forbidden the patient on a diet for low blood sugar. Even such fine additions to a normal diet as the high carbohydrate fruits, dates, figs, bananas, plums and grapes, are off limits for the hypoglycemic.*

"How can you be sure I have low blood sugar?" Ava asked.

"The way you've been eating, you couldn't escape it," I replied. "Besides, it's the only single ailment that could account for all of your numerous and varied symptoms. But if you prefer, a doctor can confirm it by giving you the six-hour Glucose Tolerance Test. After that, he'll put you on the accepted treatment for it: a high-protein, sugar-restricted diet, with frequent protein snacks during the day and before going to bed.

"It isn't hopeless," I reassured her. "Start by getting out the best pictures you have of yourself and your husband. Look at them often. Keep a mental picture of the way you looked then. Knowing that you can look like that again should give you the incentive you need to get started."

"Just telling me there's hope gives me an incentive," she said with a sigh of relief. "I was afraid I was sunk for the rest of my life in exhaustion and depression—like a mental patient or a person on a prolonged drunk."

"You *have* been on a prolonged drunk," I said, "the kind called a dry jag, or a sugar-and-starch drunk. And mental illness isn't always *mental*. In your case and many others, numerous mental aberrations that include ideas of persecution, confusion, disorderly thinking, severe depression, hallucinations and mania result from low blood sugar or a B vitamin deficiency, or both."

Ava's story had a happy ending. It wasn't easy for her to give up the sugar and starch foods she had grown to depend on. But now she had something sustaining her: the hope of regaining her mental and physical health, her looks—and her husband.

Ava's diet consisted of her choice of one or more of the complete protein foods for breakfast, lunch and dinner and protein snacks of skim milk, buttermilk, yogurt, nuts or sunflower seeds every two to three hours after meals. She was allowed her choice of fresh vegetables (except potatoes), lightly cooked or raw in salads, and all fruits except those high in carbohydrates, listed under foods that must be avoided.

She could drink any of the following: Weak tea (made with tea bag, not brewed), herb teas, caffeine-free coffee or coffee substitute (no sugar!), nonfat milk or buttermilk, and any vegetable juice or unsweetened fruit juice except prune juice and grape juice.

For dessert she could have: Fresh or unsweetened frozen or canned fruit (except those on the taboo list), cheese, unsweetened gelatin, junket (made with tablets, not the mix) and plain yogurt with choice of allowed fruit, frozen yogurt and fruit sherbet, or frozen ices made of unsweetened fruit juice.

These were to be absolutely avoided: All sweets containing sugar: candy, pie, pastries, cake, sweet rolls, custards, ice cream and sherbet (except for the unsweetened ices, yogurt and fruit sherbet listed above).

All drinks containing caffeine: coffee, strong brewed tea, cola drinks and all beverages sweetened with sugar. (If it's impossible to give up coffee for breakfast, limit it to no more than eight ounces—about a cup and a half—and keep it free of all sediment and the caffeine content down to a minimum by using the drip method of making it instead of perking or boiling.)

Potatoes, rice, figs, and grapes, as well as macaroni, spaghetti and noodles.

Wines, cordials, cocktails and beer. If you *must* have an occasional drink, make it a distilled liquor and mix it with club soda or water. (But, remember, in this instance we're dealing with a condition that prohibits sugar. In normal circumstances, my only endorsement of an alcoholic drink is a dry wine before meals as a digestive aid.)

To correct Ava's vitamin B deficiency and repair the damage to her nerves more rapidly, I recommended a cocktail made of three teaspoons of brewer's yeast, one teaspoon of desiccated liver powder and one tablespoon of lecithin granules, mixed in a glass of tomato juice and taken as a between-meal snack two or three times a day.

On this diet and with the addition of a good vitamin and mineral supplement rich in B complex, the tensions that overstimulated Ava's pancreas eased up, her nutritional deficiencies were corrected, and she lost her craving for sweets.

Another health problem, often a painful and serious threat to life itself, is also directly related to the pancreas. The victims of acute pancreatitis are admitted to hospitals in alarming numbers during the holiday season, when the pancreas is most likely to suffer an overload of sweets, starches, fats and alcohol, with the added burden of fatigue and nervous tensions that increase at this time. The overstimulated pancreas suddenly reacts—perhaps after an exceptionally heavy meal—and the racking pain of acute pancreatitis strikes. The victim is usually rushed to the hospital, where immediate and intensive care may save his life —or it may not.

Two recent cases in which the victims died involved a Los Angeles bank president and a nationally known news commentator. The finest medical treatment was still too late. The same was true of another man whose great wealth could buy anything he desired—except his health. George Vanderbilt, heir to a famous fortune, recently took his own life rather than go on suffering from the constantly recurring pain and other disabilities of chronic pancreatitis. Yet chronic pancreatitis, like diabetes, can be largely prevented by proper diet, just as it can be diet-controlled. This puts the responsibility of avoiding an acute and frequently fatal attack on the person whose life is endangered by the disease.

Here's what you can do in the majority of cases to prevent the onset of pancreatitis—or if it's too late for prevention, to keep it under control:

1. Eliminate products containing refined sugar, white flour and saturated fats from your diet. Vegetable oils and a little butter (a neutral fat) are permissible in chronic cases that are under control, *but absolutely no fats of any kind are allowed in acute cases, and no fried foods, gravies or sauces in either case.*

2. *In severe cases, avoid all concentrated sweets,* even such natural, healthful sweeteners as honey and dark molasses, which

are recommended for the normal diet. In the preventive diet, a *minimum* of natural sweeteners may be used occasionally, but not to excess. Chocolate, which contains both sugar and fats, should never be eaten.

3. Remember, protein is the food that keeps your pancreas healthy. Include one or more of the low-fat, complete proteins or high-grade vegetable proteins at every meal.

4. Let fresh fruits and vegetables and a *very moderate* amount of whole grain bread or cereal provide you with the *natural* carbohydrates you need. Avoid all refined, high-carbohydrate products.

5. Don't burden your pancreas and other organs by gorging at mealtime. The midmorning and midafternoon snacks suggested for low blood sugar will prevent the hunger that causes you to overeat.

Diseases of the pancreas are widely prevalent, yet they often go unrecognized and untreated. Medical science is very sophisticated in its knowledge about the pancreas and holds out impressive means of controlling—and curing—pancreatic disorders.

But much more research is still needed. According to the most recent report from the Hypoglycemia Foundation, science is just beginning to "lift the lid on the critical part that the elusive enzymes play in the whole picture." Many diabetics improve dramatically, without insulin or oral medication, on the low blood sugar diet for hypoglycemics. Their research also found that many cases of heart disease can be avoided by following the same sugar-restricted diet.

A diet high in sugar and starch has recently been blamed for still another painful disease. Writing in the *British Medical Journal* (July, 1966), Dr. T. L. Cleave, former surgeon-captain of Great Britain's Royal Navy, gives evidence that refined carbohydrates are responsible for the intestinal changes that cause *diverticulitis,* the formation and inflammation of tiny pouches upon a weakened intestinal wall.

Dr. Cleave's research was in opposition to the long-held theory that this severe and painful condition of the colon (often requiring surgery as a last resort) eventually "just happens" to at least twenty percent of everyone over forty! Dr. Cleave and Dr. G. D. Campbell discovered two simple but significant facts that you can use for your own protection:

1. The victims of diverticulitis were always among those eating excessive amounts of white flour and sugar products. The majority of them were overweight.
2. *Persons of normal weight who ate a diet that omitted refined carbohydrates simply did not get diverticulitis!*

Drs. Cleave and Campbell found the disease nonexistent in countries where "civilized" and devitalized carbohydrates were unknown. They advise for success in "the prevention and arrest of the disease, *a very considerable restoration of the carbohydrates to their natural unrefined state.*" But until that happens on a national scale, protect your own health by eating only the unrefined, natural sugar and starch foods that have already been recommended.

The diseases that are either caused or made worse by refined carbohydrates and saturated fats are too numerous to list in one chapter. And each year of research adds new and surprising names to the list. Arthritis is one of them. The four major—and avoidable—factors that can trigger destructive changes in the joints are: starvation of the tissues, retention of toxins, infections and chemical imbalance.

Infection causes an imbalance in the body chemistry that is frequently responsible for arthritis. Yet even after the source of infection (such as tonsils or teeth) is removed, the arthritis remains.

Mental and emotional strain and conditions that interfere with the circulation can cause bouts with arthritis that may be only temporary.

But one of the major causes of arthritis, an inadequate and unbalanced diet, is often overlooked. Poor nutrition causes a chemical imbalance and starves the tissues, and both these conditions invite the disease. Moreover, improper diet weakens the body's ability to protect itself and makes it powerless to rebuild its cells and thereby avoid further degeneration and permanent damage to the tissues.

A former arthritic who is an authority on degenerative diseases, Dr. Melvin E. Page, director of the Page Foundation, St. Petersburg, Florida, says, "In my clinic practice it has been found that the diets of arthritics are preponderantly carbohydrate and deficient in trace minerals. Usually a deficiency of B vitamins is found." Dr. Page emphasizes the fact that eating sugar violates the fundamental rules of health, and he verifies my own conviction when he says, "Refined sugar and white flour are the most common and the most harmful elements in our diet."

Reporting on the successful treatment of rheumatoid, osteo and mixed arthritic cases, Dr. Charles A. Brusch, medical director, Brusch Medical Center, Cambridge, Massachusetts, also stressed the value of *"complete abstinence from white sugar plus a wholesome diet."* (My italics) The treatment he recommends is to coordinate these factors:

1. A wholesome diet, free from refined food.
2. Control of water and fluid intake.
3. One tablespoon of cod-liver oil given daily in two tablespoons of orange juice or milk, preferably five hours after eating or on an empty stomach. (Diabetics and heart patients were the exceptions who were given it only twice a week.)

The second factor, control of water and fluid intake, might require supervision, but the other two are well within your control. And you don't have to have arthritis to benefit from them.

We have seen repeatedly how following sound nutritional principles can protect health, youth, and life. To insure the benefits of proper diet, however, the digestive system must be kept in good working order. The stomach and the intestines are delicate mechanisms and should not be strained or overloaded. In the following chapter we will discuss how the digestive system functions and what you must do to keep it running smoothly.

9

How to Keep Your "Food Factory" in Order

Your human food factory can develop "labor troubles" just as other manufacturing plants do. Yet it's a factory capable of giving a lifetime of efficient service if you don't overload it, or clog the machinery with waste products, and if you supply the proper fuel to keep it running smoothly.

Your mouth, like the opening of a furnace, takes in fuel necessary to run the factory. It's also in your mouth that digestion begins. When you clog the digestive machinery with improper fuel or allow outside influences to interfere with it, you start a chain reaction of labor troubles in your human food factory. Indigestion and constipation are the ringleaders, organizing the strikes and marshaling protest marchers that rumble and grumble up and down the colon. So it's time we found out more about the damage these troublemakers cause and what can be done to prevent it.

Indigestion and Constipation

"Digestion is a delicate biochemical process," wrote Dr. Boris Sokoloff in *The Civilized Diseases*. "The colon, more than any other organ, seems *poorly* adjusted to civilized life. It is easily affected by anything associated with our modern way of living: *improper food, nervous strain, fatigue—affect the colon immediately.*" (My italics)

I thought of that truism as I watched popular singer Al Henshaw gulp several antacid tablets after a meal he had wolfed down almost as fast as he swallowed the pills.

"Nervous indigestion," he explained, half-apologetically, "and an acid stomach."

"What do you mean, an 'acid stomach'?" I asked.

"Well—just an acid condition—or maybe hyperacidity."

"Yes, I know," I said. "I hear hundreds of complaints of 'acid stomach,' and all of them are just as vague as yours." Then I told him of a few of the things he should know before doctoring himself for what he called an acid stomach.

"First, your stomach *has* to be acid, or you can't digest protein and other fibrous foods. Second, as you grow older, the acidity of the stomach decreases. About ninety percent of people in their second forty years have *too little acid* to digest and absorb the protein foods they must have to keep their health and youthful energy."

"I'm sure losing mine," Al said.

"Instead of swallowing those pills by the dozen, you should find out whether you need *more* acid instead of less to aid your digestion," I advised. "And while you're about it, have an examination to discover whether you actually *have* indigestion—"

"I know I have," he interrupted.

"You know you have stomach pains that you *think* are caused by indigestion," I said, "and I hope they are."

"It's just nervous indigestion," Al insisted. "I've had it for years, but it kicks up worse when I'm tired, worried and under pressure, or eat when I'm nervous, which is most of the time."

These facts seemed to indicate that Al's pain was not caused by an organic disease. But I still recommended an examination to rule out entirely any such possibility. "Acid stomach" and "nervous indigestion" are easy labels. Far too many persons use them to describe any kind of upper abdominal pain, without bothering to find out whether or not it results from a minor cause or a major illness, such as coronary thrombosis or cancer of the stomach. Peptic ulcer, a bad appendix and gall bladder disorders are other conditions that are often self-diagnosed as "indigestion."

Disturbances of the stomach and intestines are among the most frequent causes of pain in the over-forty age group. Records of examinations reveal that in more than fifty percent of these cases there is no organic disease. However, to be safe, find out for sure. Don't depend on your own diagnosis.

Some months later Al Henshaw and I were having dinner again. But this time he sipped a glass of dry wine before dinner instead of his usual double martinis. He sat relaxed, eating slowly, enjoying his broiled steak, steamed asparagus, fresh tomatoes and watercress topped wth yogurt.

"It's a funny thing," he went on, "since I've been relaxing more and eating as you advised, including yogurt and buttermilk, I've stopped getting heartburn, stomach pains and the acid taste in my mouth."

It would have taken more time than either of us had to give Al a step-by-step account of his digestive processes, but there were a few facts that I thought he would like to know.

"Your gastrointestinal tract is governed by your involuntary nervous system," I told him. "One set of nerves contracts the musculature of the digestive organs, while another set promotes its relaxation. When the two sets of nerves get out of balance you get what you've been calling nervous, or acid, indigestion."

"But what got mine out of balance?" he asked.

"*You* did," I said, "by your consistently poor eating habits: by eating the wrong food, by eating too fast, by overeating at any time, but especially when you were overtired and during emotional disturbances, which in your case were frequent."

Digestion involves a complex interplay of nerves, muscles, chemicals and bacteria, coupled with precise meshing of signals. When something goes wrong with this complex interplay—and complex it is, as you'll learn in the enzyme chapter—whether from physical, emotional or nutritional failure, digestive disorders occur. Because of "indigestion," each year Americans lose a total of some 50,000,000 working days, with a loss to industry of more than $250,000,000. Only respiratory diseases (mostly colds and flu) have the dubious distinction of topping that record.

In addition to his improved diet, better habits of relaxation, effective use of the enzyme activators and avoidance of the inhibitors, Al found these suggestions helpful:

1. Eat leisurely and chew well to give the salivary enzymes a chance to mix with food. But don't take the pleasure out of eating by believing it's necessary to chew each mouthful a stipulated number of times, because it isn't. Food digests better when it's *enjoyed.*

2. Don't be an air swallower. Air is for breathing, not gulping. Yet many high-strung people hastily gulp their food and beverages, taking in large quantities of air at the same time. Gum chewers are often air gulpers, too. When your stomach is filled with air, how else can it feel except bloated?

It may surprise you to know that digestive functions of older persons differ very little from those of the young. But here are some of the things to watch out for as you grow older:

1. *Digestion can be seriously retarded as enzymes grow fewer and weaker with the passing years.* You'll learn this and what to do about it in the next chapter.

2. *The ability to withstand abuse and strain decreases.* Overeating is among the worst forms of abuse. Don't burden your stomach and stretch its capacity by overloading it with too much food, especially with fat-and-carbohydrate-heavy meals. For many people, eating smaller, more frequent meals can be helpful. If there are foods you can't tolerate, by this time you should know what they are and be wise enough *not* to eat them. There is such a wide and delicious variety of foods you *can* eat without distress that you shouldn't really miss those that give you trouble. But read on, and you'll see it may not be *what* you eat that causes indigestion, but how you feel when you eat it.

3. *At any age, fatigue and tension interfere with digestion. So do worry, anger, fear, self-pity, defeatism and similar negative*

emotions. Both physical and mental strain are more detrimental to the older person, who has less ability to bounce back from them. Dr. Walter Alvarez of the Mayo Clinic, famous specialist in gastrointestinal disorders, stated, "The commonest causes of 'nervous indigestion' are fatigue, worry, hypersensitiveness and insomnia."

4. *As noted before, acidity of the stomach tends to decline as you grow older.* In the following pages we will discuss the various means of restoring normal acidity.

Aging and Your Acid Balance

You will learn a good deal about digestion in the chapter on enzymes, including the fact that your stomach must be acid to digest protein foods which renew and rebuild your body's cells. So, by simple logic, the reverse is true—an alkaline stomach prevents good digestion, and aging is speeded up.

It was in experiments made by Dr. George A. Wilson that the striking parallel between alkalinity and aging was demonstrated. Testing many men and women in their eighties, he found that those with an acid dominance were healthy, alert and young for their age. Those with an alkaline dominance were not. With a few variations, his recommendations for correcting overalkalinity and improving the acid balance are the same as mine. Here is a combination of his overall plan, with my expansions and additions:

1. Eat properly balanced meals. (This book and all my others tell you how.)

2. Avoid devitalized starches and sweets (those made with white flour and refined sugar).

3. Live a balanced life, which includes work, rest, relaxation and exercise.

4. Build up resistance to unavoidable stresses by "rolling with the punches." Also by including plenty of nerve-calming calcium and vitamin-B-rich foods and supplements in your diet.

5. Use acidizing aids. My favorite natural acid restorers are apple cider vinegar and the valuable lactic-acid foods, like

yogurt and buttermilk, which can substitute (at least in part) for hydrochloric acid.

Constipation

In her book *Ageless Youth,* Dr. Charlotte West claims that constipation is too often ignored when it doesn't give rise to actual pain. "It does give rise to a vast amount of health and beauty defects," she says. "Who can be attractive with an offensive breath, a muddy skin, dull eyes, a listless manner and dullness of mind?"

Who, indeed? No one can surmount such barriers to charm. Yet the person who allows constipation to become habitual may suffer not only from these defects, but from far more serious afflictions.

Both indigestion and constipation are ailments of the digestive tract. There is a prevalent misconception that indigestion affects only the stomach and constipation only the intestinal tract. The two subjects are inseparable; what affects one is related to the other. The poor eating habits and lack of enzymes that prevent digestion can cause constipation. So can a number of other bad habits and emotional conditions that also trigger indigestion. Habitual constipation may indicate the need for psychological readjustment. Or it may be the symptom of an organic disease.

There are several forms of constipation. The most common is *atonic* constipation, in which the large intestine and abdominal muscles lose "tone." It can be caused by any or all of the following:

1. Postponing the urge to go to stool—or ignoring it completely until the "signal corps" quits functioning.

Remedy: Establish regular bowel habits at a certain time each day until this becomes routine, which it will if you are persistent and allow nothing to interfere or cause postponement.

2. Inadequate intake of fluids.

Remedy: Drink more water, at least six glasses or more between meals. Water helps cleanse and flush impurities from the body. It prevents dehydration, which may occur in anyone, but especially in older people.

3. High-carbohydrate diets.

Remedy: Avoid the soft, refined diet that consists largely of white flour and refined sugar products. Such food leaves no residue for excretion. Cut down on bread, which can cause constipation, although raw wheat does not. The raw seed contains enzymes that aid digestion and promote elimination. Eat the high-protein, enzyme-rich foods recommended in Chapter 10.

4. Lack of physical activity.

Remedy: Get off your seat and on your feet as much as possible. Walking is good. The familiar deep-knee bends or squatting exercise, if done every day, will strengthen abdominal muscles. So will pulling in your abdominal muscles as far as you can and holding them tightly for a count of twenty or until the tensed muscles begin to quiver. If done as little as two minutes a day, this exercise will flatten the abdomen, strengthen and tone the muscles.

5. The cathartic and laxative habit.

Remedy: Break the habit! The dependence on laxatives can produce secondary constipation. Rely on nature's call and natural foods and supplements—especially those rich in B vitamins—not drugs. You can continue eating natural foods, with good results, for a lifetime.

If you feel you *must* occasionally depend on something as you're forming new health habits, there are a few mild activators containing laxative herbs that can be used when absolutely necessary. But these should be only occasional aids to help you "taper off" as you break the laxative habit.

Best Laxative Foods

Blackstrap molasses: A tablespoonful taken at night is a fine natural laxative, besides being rich in B vitamins, iron, calcium and other minerals. It may be taken straight, stirred into a glass of water, or mixed with milk. (The calcium in both the milk and molasses make this combination an excellent sleep inducer.) And just as you would after eating any concentrated sweet, brush your teeth or rinse your mouth afterward.

Honey: Another good natural laxative, but milder than molasses. For an in-between strength, try mixing half honey and half molasses.

Flaxseed: In *atonic* constipation, two or three tablespoons of flaxseed can be chewed at intervals during the day for good results. Or the meal may be cooked in cereal, sprinkled over cereals and salads, or mixed with liquids. If mixed with liquid, drink at once before the mixture thickens.

Lubricating oils: Add two or three tablespoons of safflower, sunflower, sesame, soybean or corn oil to your diet each day, not only to "lubricate the machinery," but for extra nutritional benefits that are discussed elsewhere in this book. Mix them with lemon juice or cider vinegar for a salad dressing. Take them by the spoonful if you like. *Never* use mineral oil, as it robs the body of two valuable minerals—calcium and phosphorous—and of vitamins A, D and E.

Brewer's yeast, wheat germ, sprouted grains: Because of their high vitamin B content, these foods keep the muscles of the intestinal tract from becoming weak and prolapsed. They help promote normal elimination.

Yogurt: The best friend your intestinal tract ever had! Yogurt manufactures B vitamins necessary to keep it clean, healthy and vigorous. By means of lactic acid, yogurt increases the "friendly" intestinal bacteria, which fight hostile germs that invade the colon.

When the friendly bacteria decrease in number—they can be destroyed by antibiotics and washed away by laxatives—the enemy bacteria move in. Unless they are outnumbered and outfought by our friendly protectors, constipation, with its many problems, gains a strong foothold. More and more doctors are recommending yogurt to restore the friendly bacteria in patients who have taken antibiotics. Dr. Boris Sokoloff is convinced that we should have at least 100,000,000,000 of these friendly bacilli a day. That sounds like an incredible number, but eating one or two cups of yogurt a day will provide approximately that amount.

Spastic Constipation and Colitis

The spastic colon is a nervous disorder, a functional disturbance of the bowels, in which irregular spasms and relaxations of the muscular wall of the intestine take the place of normal, coordinated contractions. In colitis, there may be alternating constipation and diarrhea, gas formation and abdominal pain. Excessive smoking and too much coffee can contribute to the trouble. But the spastic condition of the bowels results from the same emotional disturbances that cause indigestion: fatigue, overwork, worry, anxiety and tension.

Foods rich in calcium, magnesium, B vitamins and lecithin improve the nerves, helping them respond normally, instead of overreacting to disturbing factors. Less roughage in the diet is usually indicated but a big part of the treatment must be directed toward correcting the environment and conditions that cause the trouble and toward improving the general health, nerves and entire personality of the patient so his reactions to outside influences will not cause the disturbed innervation of the bowels.

Your human food factory is more sensitive and complex than any manmade piece of machinery you own. Yet it's also the most durable and efficient. Keep it running smoothly with a minimum of friction, feed it the proper fuel, don't overload it or clog up the works, and it will last a lifetime without breaking down, cracking up or wearing out!

Digestion, metabolism and all vital bodily processes are controlled by enzymes. These enzymes are supplied both in food and by the body. In the next chapter, we will discuss how the enzyme system works and how its optimal functioning vitalizes the body and promotes longer life.

10

The Antiaging Power of Enzymes

A Nobel Prize winner, Dr. James B. Sumner of Cornell University, called enzymes the secret of life. And according to extensive experiments and research, that's *just* what they are! Without enzymes, there would be no plant, animal or human life. Seeds would fail to sprout. You would never have been born. And if you have neurotic days when you wish you hadn't, that, too, can be due to a lack of enzymes.

Dr. Sumner claims that when you start losing vitality and getting that fortyish feeling, it's because the enzymes in your body grow fewer and weaker as you grow older. This fact was verified in a report ("Status of Food Enzymes in Digestion and Metabolism") by Edward Howell which explained how the body, *when it was not given sufficient raw materials from raw foods,* grew tired and produced fewer and weaker enzymes with each passing year. The importance of raw fruits and vegetables has been emphasized in all my writings. But it takes a chapter on enzymes to give some of the reasons that are not commonly known.

When your enzymes grow weak and feeble, so do you. Just as enzyme-deficient plant life and insect life dries and shrivels, the human body, deprived of enzymes, becomes weak. Face and body undergo the sagging, withering process we associate with aging. The description sounds like a protein deficiency, and in effect, it is. Only worse. A lack of enzymes can create a deficiency of *all* the nutrients. Without enzyme action, the food you eat is not digested and absorbed. When this occurs, you can suffer from malnutrition, deficiency diseases and early aging following the best diet in the world.

Enzymes direct all of the chemical reactions that go on in your billions of cells. They have been called "chemical tools" that convert protein and other nutrients into the only form of nourishment your cells can use. An important part of their job is to split every bite of food you eat into microscopic fragments that can be absorbed through the intestinal wall.

But what are enzymes, actually? Let dancer Kathryn Murray give the first clue. When in her fifties, she was asked how she and Arthur managed to put in such long hours and still retain their incredibly youthful energy. She gave credit to a good diet that consisted of plenty of lean meat, eggs, green salads, fresh vegetables and fruits. "Whatever makes the juices flow," is the way she put it. She probably didn't know that she was speaking of enzymes, but that's what they are—internal juices. The food the dancing Murrays ate and their extreme physical activity combined to stimulate that flow and to provide what's called a favorable environment for enzyme production.

Enzymologists tell us our bodies contain many millions of each type of enzyme. There are more than 700 different types, each performing a separate task. They fall into two general classifications:

1. *Endogenous enzymes, produced within your own cells and tissues.* They can be stimulated to a more active production, as you will learn.

2. *Exogenous enzymes, obtained through the food you eat.* Among the best sources of *exogenous* enzymes are raw fresh fruits and vegetables, plus the other foods listed beginning on page 49.

Carlson Wade in his book *Help Your Health Through Enzymes* calls these internal juices "a built-in fountain of youth," and believes they may be the "secret key" to health and a longer youth.

"Enzymes are part of all living things, from the cells in a weed to the cells in your brain," he says. ". . . *All bodily processes, mental and physical, healing and maintenance, are ruled by enzymes, those substances that have the power to rejuvenate an entire being.*" (My italics)

The different types of enzymes have their own specific jobs to do, and one type never pinch-hits for another. If your protein-digesting enzymes are too few and feeble to do their work, the protein you eat just won't be broken down into usable form. The enzymes that break down fats and starches will not aid the digestion of protein—even if your life depends upon it, which it might! *Without the complex series of enzymatic actions and reactions, there would be no digestion, and it would be impossible for the food you eat to nourish your body cells.*

It isn't necessary for you to know the names and functions of all the enzymes. But to give you a general knowledge of them, here are a few of the better-known ones, with the places they are found, the type of food they work on and what they change food into for cell nourishment:

Found in the mouth: Ptyalin.

Ptyalin is a salivary enzyme that acts upon starches and sugars, breaking them down into dextrins. To get the full benefit of this first step in digesting carbohydrates, the mouth should be alkaline and all sugar and starch foods should be chewed thoroughly to blend with ptyalin.

Found in the stomach: Pepsin, rennin, lipase.

Pepsin is a most vital digestive enzyme. It acts upon proteins, splitting them into preotoses and peptones to make usable amino acids. When pepsin is lacking, your body is unable to use protein, and even on a high-protein diet, you will suffer a deficiency.

Rennin acts on milk and other dairy foods, changing their protein (casein) into a usable form called paracasein and releasing valuable minerals for the body's use.

In addition to proteins and vitamins, the normal functioning and life of your cells require iron, calcium, magnesium, zinc, cobalt, copper, manganese and other trace minerals, some of which are contained in enzymes themselves and all of which are activated by them.

Lipase is a fat-splitting enzyme that partially digests fats in the stomach before the job is finally completed in the small intestine. Lipase is a product of the "enzyme factory" of the pancreas. This large gland back of the stomach manufactures a number of specialized enzymes that travel through a duct to reach the digestive system.

Found in the small intestine: Steapsin, trypsin, erepsin, rennin, amylopsin, invertase, maltase, lactase, and some others.

Steapsin acts upon fats already partially digested by lipase and finishes changing them into fatty acids and glycerol.

Trypsin takes over proteins after their initial splitting by pepsin, changing them into peptides, which are then changed to amino acids.

Erepsin uses still another sleight-of-enzyme trick on protein, changing peptides to amino acids.

Rennin is present in the intestine as it is in the stomach, ready to complete the job of changing the casein of milk products into usable paracasein.

Amylopsin breaks down starch, changing it to glucose.

Invertase does the same with sugar, and the result is glucose and fructose. (Invertase can break down 1,000,000 times its own weight in sugar!)

Maltase changes maltose into dextrins.

Lactase has the job of converting milk sugar (lactose) into glucose and galactose.

These are just a few examples of the enzymes that transform the food you eat into substances your body must have. But enzymes do more than *prevent* disease and the shortening of your youth and life. Medical science is continually discovering new ways of using them to fight existing diseases.

The Healing Power of Enzymes

Trypsin, efficient in breaking down protein, is being used to dissolve blood clots, a procedure that comes naturally to it, since clots consist partly of protein substances. New York's Bellevue Hospital has used it extensively in the treatment of leg blood clots (thrombophlebitis), and its value was confirmed at a conference held at the New York Academy of Sciences.

Of special interest to women is a report made on bromelin, an enzyme found in pineapple stems and isolated by Dr. Ralph Heinicke of the University of Minnesota. Bromelin has been found effective in relieving menstrual pains and in easing difficult childbirth. Further tests should prove it useful in some problems of the menopause.

According to Dr. J. L. Blonstein, physician for the Amateur Boxing Association of London, black eyes, blood clots, broken-down tissues, bruises, abrasions, cuts and swellings can be successfully treated by a combination of two enzymes, streptokinase and streptodornase. With this enzyme treatment, Dr. Blonstein reported to the London *Times,* a fifty percent reduction of bruises and abrasions and a fifteen percent reduction of blood swellings occurred, and healing took only one-fourth to one-half as long as it normally did.

Other enzymes have proved their healing power in treating afflictions that range from the minor to the catastrophic. Among the relatively minor ones is one reported by Dr. John C. Houck of Children's Hospital Research Foundation in Washington, D. C. An enzyme called procollagenase has proved effective in preventing the formation of scar tissue, and in literally dissolving or erasing scars that already exist. Again enzymes are doing what comes naturally to them, as scars develop from a form of collagen, a fibrous protein.

Urease was isolated from jack beans by Dr. James B. Sumner, mentioned at the beginning of this chapter. Urease breaks down urea, a substance formed in the liver and transported to the kidneys by the bloodstream. If not broken down by urease and passed from the body, urea can create a toxic condition.

As enzyme research broadens, important breakthroughs continue to make news. Papain, an enzyme from the tropical fruit papaya, is best known as a digestive aid. A Chicago orthopedic surgeon, Dr. Lyman Smith, also holds out great hopes for it in slipped disk therapy. Testing papain on animals by injecting it into the nucleus of the disk, Dr. Lyman reported that this papaya enzyme dissolved the nucleus and, by eliminating pressure, relieved the pain.

Papain offers relief for many ailments, reports Dr. Philip Pollack in *Current Therapeutic Research.* In forty-nine patients given papain, Dr. Pollack found it effective in treating such diverse conditions as skin allergies, bedsores, hemorrhoids, heart disease.

The American Chemical Society, at an annual meeting in Atlantic City, New Jersey, reported that cholesterol has been dissolved in the arteries of animals by the enzyme elastase. Research is now under way to see if enzymes will reduce excess cholesterol and dissolve deposits in human arteries. If successful, it would indicate means of controlling two killer diseases, strokes and coronary thrombosis.

Parkinson's disease, a disabling disease that afflicts 1,000,000 or more Americans, is responding effectively, though so far only temporarily, to treatment with extracted enzymes. A Canadian friend of mine, Pierre LeMoyne, was stricken with this disease and was changed from a youthful, robust fifty to a feeble, quivering old man. I knew that somehow he must be given hope to go on—not false hope, but belief in a possible cure based on the progress being made.

I asked him whether he had heard of the work being done on Parkinson's disease by doctors and researchers at the University of Montreal, and he replied with amazement that he didn't know anything *could* be done.

"They've been treating the disease with enzymes," I explained, "and the American Academy of Neurology has a report that tells of the remarkable results they've had."

"Then why isn't the treatment available to me?" he asked. I explained that patients treated with enzymes have shown tremendous improvement, but so far, it's been only temporary.

"What's the chance that this will lead to a permanent cure?" he asked.

"Scientists are working on it," I said. "At the University of Montreal they found that the brains of patients with Parkinson's disease show an abnormally low concentration of two related chemicals, dopamine and sorotonia. They theorized that this deficiency might be caused by a lack of certain enzymes. Their theory led to the present treatment with extracted enzymes. The patients treated show an amazing improvement. At this stage of research the results are only temporary—but the research continues."

Then I told him how to give himself an enzyme treatment with every meal. Not a treatment for specific diseases, such as the one he had. For that you must have the isolated enzymes given by injection, or in a highly concentrated oral form. Wherever fresh, raw fruits and vegetables and natural, unprocessed foods are available, I told Pierre, almost everyone can gain the health benefits of daily enzyme treatments. It's a matter of knowing what foods contain them. It is also important to avoid factors that inhibit enzyme action.

Foods That Supply Your Daily Enzymes

1. *Fresh Raw Fruits and Vegetables*

For the enzyme way to better health and a longer youth, have *at least one fresh, raw fruit or vegetable at each meal.* They are rich sources of enzymes, vitamins and minerals. Some of the vitamins in them act as coenzymes that help spark enzymatic action. And just as enzymes are necessary to release and utilize the minerals in these and other foods, so are minerals essential aids to enzymes in carrying out their work.

One mineral, magnesium, acts as a coenzyme in the building of protein. There is a mutual-dependence relationship between enzymes and other minerals. Here are just a few examples:

Enzymes need iron to help bring about oxidative reactions, to carry oxygen to all parts of your body, including your brain, and to help form protein compounds of nucleic acid for your cells.

Iodine is needed to help enzymes bring about glandular action. Your thyroid gland is dependent upon enzymes to spark the process before it can secrete thyroxin. This makes enzymes partly responsible for the rate of your mental processes. The activity of your brain depends to a large extent upon your thyroid and its hormone secretion, thyroxin—which in turn depend upon enzymes to activate *them.*

This is just a small sample to give you an idea of the countless actions, reactions and interactions in which enzymes are involved. But the important thing to remember is that a deficiency in a single enzyme, vitamin or mineral (and, of course, protein) can impair your health. Serious deficiencies in any or all of them can endanger your life. Cooking (especially at high heat) destroys most enzymes and many vitamins. So, as often as you can, eat raw fruits and vegetables. If you feel you *must* cook some vegetables, see my book, *Cook Right—Live Longer,* and learn how to avoid nutricide in your kitchen.

2. *Protein Foods*

Enzymes and proteins work together to maintain your health and youthful vitality and to restore them when they slip away because of faulty nutrition.

You already know the complete proteins on which your daily meals should be based (see Chapter 5). Just as a reminder, you should have one or more of them at each meal, if at all possible. And if not, be sure to substitute one or more of the other high-quality proteins. Enzymes themselves are proteins. Some of the amino acids they make from protein to nourish your body are needed for their own sustenance. Only *you* can supply the vital needs of your cells and enzymes for amino acids by providing them with plenty of high-grade protein each day.

3. *Some Supercharged Enzyme Foods*

Yogurt: This almost-perfect food is a rich source of enzymes that aid digestion, the absorption of protein, calcium and other nutrients, and help set up a miniature "factory" that manufactures B vitamins in your body. These and its other plus qualities give yogurt an extra advantage: It's a matter of record that in countries such as Bulgaria where it's eaten regularly, people stay young and vital longer. (For more on yogurt, including how to make it and yogurt recipes from all over the world, see my book *Cook Right–Live Longer.*)

Brewer's yeast: Yeast cells are "living food" for enzymes–and for humans. For years I have recommended brewer's yeast as a potent and highly concentrated source of many nutrients, especially the entire family of B vitamins. Brewer's yeast serves a threefold purpose in the care and feeding of enzymes:

1. It "feeds" them.
2. It activates them.
3. It's a superior source of enzyme-producing agents.

Wheat germ: Raw wheat germ is, like brewer's yeast, a fine source of B vitamins, protein and other nutrients that nourish and activate enzymes and enable them to carry out their work. All raw grains contain enzymes, which grinding doesn't destroy but which the heat of cooking does. If you'd like to know how to prepare wheat and other grains with a minimum of enzyme loss, or if you're interested in grinding your own, again I refer you to my book *Cook Right–Live Longer.*

Sprouts: Sprouted legumes and grains contain a high concentration of enzymes, vitamins, minerals, and an additional wonder-working element, a root auxin (plant hormone) that aids enzymes and amino acids in producing youthful cells and renewing old ones.

Mung bean sprouts are available in many supermarkets in the fresh produce department. Or you can sprout your own. There are several books that will tell you how, including–if you'll pardon the repetition!–my own *Cook Right–Live Longer.*

Papaya: This tropical fruit, available now in most large supermarkets, is rich in the enzyme papain, which aids digestion and helps break down protein into amino acids. Like all fresh, raw fruits, it contains many vitamins, minerals and enzymes. But it's especially acclaimed for its high papain content. When the fresh fruit is not available, try your health food store for canned papaya slices, papaya pulp, and unsweetened papaya juice. (Digestive enzymes containing papain are available in tablet form.)

Nuts and seeds: All *raw* seeds and nuts are rich in enzymes. Be sure to get them *un*toasted, *un*roasted and *un*processed. Buy nuts in the shell whenever possible. Sunflower seeds are tedious to shell, so for convenience, health food stores sell the raw, shelled (dehusked) seeds. Their other valuable nutrients will be discussed in a later chapter.

Peanut and almond butter: Made of raw nuts and not homogenized, these two concentrated foods are rich sources of enzymes, amino acids, vitamins, minerals. They are available in health food stores and some markets. You can make your own with raw nuts of your choice, a food grinder and safflower oil (enough to give it the consistency you like). Add a little sea salt to individual taste.

Here is my recipe for an enzyme pickup nutritious enough for a meal on days when time doesn't permit a leisurely breakfast or luncheon. (For a between-meal pickup, have smaller portions.)

THE LELORD KORDEL ENZYME BOOSTER

Blend together one cup of yogurt, one cup of fresh papaya, orange or pineapple juice, one-third cup of sunflower seeds, three tablespoons of wheat germ and one of brewer's yeast. If desired, sweeten with honey. (Sometimes I add a few almonds, some fresh berries and a raw egg yolk for extra enzymes and other nutritive benefits.)

Enzyme Inhibitors to Avoid

Tension and fatigue: Whenever possible, take a few minutes to rest and relax before meals.

Unpleasant surroundings, arguments at the table and discussions of bad news inhibit enzyme action. If you *must* argue or view the world's situation (and your own) with alarm, do it between meals.

Gulping large amounts of liquids with meals: Washing food down with water or other beverages dilutes and weakens the enzyme flow. Enzymes need water, but don't *drown* them at mealtime.

Lack of oxygen and exercise: Your enzymes need oxygenation, so give it to them—and to yourself. It's easy to do. If you're a shallow breather (most women are), practice deep, abdominal breathing as you walk or exercise in the fresh air or before an open window until it comes naturally to you. The oxygen you take in enables your body, with the aid of enzymes as chemical tools, to burn carbohydrates and other digested foods to produce energy. If the air you breathe is cold, dry or debris-laden, a specialized enzyme, lysozyme, warms, humidifies and filters it for you.

Enzyme Activators

To stimulate enzyme action, start each meal with one of these: fresh, raw fruit, a raw-vegetable salad, a cup of meat or vegetable broth or a glass of dry wine (diluted with water). All of them are rich in certain extractive substances that prepare your stomach for the meal to follow. They do this by stimulating the cells in the lower stomach to produce greater quantities of the hormone secretin which, in a series of actions and reactions, results in a flow into the stomach of a most vital digestive enzyme, hydrochloric acid.

Your stomach is acid or should be—no matter what you think to the contrary. Or how you may complain of "acid stomach"! In an alkaline environment, the enzymes in your stomach are unable to function. Without hydrochloric acid, the protein and iron in your food are not absorbed and converted to the form essential for your body's use.

As you grow older the flow of hydrochloric acid may decrease. If so, your doctor will recommend hydrochloric acid tablets or liquid or "something sour" eaten with protein foods. My own recommendation for restoring stomach acid and promoting protein absorption is this natural way that also includes other health benefits: one tablespoon of apple cider vinegar in a glass of water each morning before breakfast and one teaspoon in water during or after other protein meals.

If you are beginning to feel the effects of aging, don't inhibit the enzymes you have left by destructive worrying when you can take positive steps to remedy the condition. First, you can create a favorable enzyme environment. This means making sure your mouth is kept alkaline and your stomach acid so your enzymes will have the right medium in which to work. It also means avoiding the enzyme inhibitors. Next, you can replenish your supply of food enzymes each day by giving your body sufficient raw materials from raw foods. You will see how your body responds by giving you better health, more vitality and a longer-lasting youth.

11

Habits That Make You Look Older and Age Faster

Your habits, depending upon whether they are good or bad, can make a difference not only in how young you look but in how long you live.

An old Spanish proverb tells us, "Habits are at first cobwebs, then cables." Some habits are simply acquired mannerisms that make you look older without affecting your health. These are the harmless, cobweb habits that are easy to break if you recognize them and start resisting them early.

The dangerous habits are those that gradually tighten their cablelike hold on you until, before you realize it, they become necessities. By that time their grip on you is so strong that you may need help to break them. When a habit becomes a crutch to lean on, a necessity that leads to harmful excesses, the warning signal, DANGER—POTENTIAL KILLER! is already overdue.

We'll begin with some of the harmless and comparatively easily broken cobweb habits before tackling the dangerous variety. Since man is a creature of habit, breaking a few of the easy ones first helps him form a good one—*the habit of breaking habits.* And that's one he will need in his attempt to free himself from the imprisoning bonds of the cable habits.

Cobweb Habits

Most of the cobweb habits are harmless—if you consider anything "harmless" that makes you look older than you should! —and all of them do.

Nose Wrinkling: This is an overworked feminine habit. It can be cute in a child and rather charming in a young girl. But unless the habit is broken early, the charming crinkles all too soon develop into deep, aging wrinkles.

If you're over fifteen and wrinkle your nose like a bunny when you smile, look closely and you'll see that fine lines are already beginning to etch themselves on the crinkly sides of your nose, lines that become unsightly grooves by the time you're thirty. If you're over thirty, lots of lubrication and light massage will soften the furrows, but only breaking the habit will prevent their returning and deepening.

To show a young nose-wrinkling niece of mine what was happening to her, I presented her with a large magnifying mirror. When she saw the magnified results of her mannerism, she gasped, "I've got a wrinkled thumb on my face!" Her metaphor was mixed, but the image gave her the incentive she needed to break the habit and get rid of the crinkles.

Mouth Puckering: Both men and women are guilty of this wrinkle-forming habit, which hasn't looked good on them since they were babies puckering up to cry. I can think of only one good excuse for puckering up the lips, though even this has its limitations. "Who wants to kiss a prune?" is the way my teen-age daughter put it. "Soft, smooth lips are in—puckering is definitely *out.*"

Do you purse your mouth as though you had a drawstring in it when you concentrate, are displeased, tense or frustrated? If you do, watch out! It's an aging mannerism, more noticeable among elderly persons, but it can start while you're young. So every time you feel a pucker coming on, smooth out the creases and avoid prune lips by deliberately relaxing those tightened muscles. A smile or a yawn will do it.

What if you aren't a mouth purser, yet the puckers are there for no discernible reason? A network of wrinkles gathered around your mouth, with cracks and splits at the corners that are slow to heal. Puckered lines that spread out from the lips, sometimes extending almost to the nose, and corners of the mouth that crack—are two of the many disfigurements caused by a deficiency of riboflavin, one of the B vitamins. So you can see that poor nutritional habits age you rapidly unless they are broken and replaced with good ones.

Jaw Jutting and Mouth Clamping: These go-together habits not only make you look old, they advertise your date of birth, since it's the older age group that has a monopoly on them. While typically masculine, a surprising number of women acquire these mannerisms, particularly those who tend to develop mannish characteristics as they grow older. You can avoid these and other aging mannerisms and nervous grimaces by being alert to early tendencies. Don't allow even one to sneak up on you. If it does, correct it before the habit is set.

Mugwump Habits

The Spanish proverb didn't mention mugwump habits. It's what I call those that are in between the cobwebs and cables. You remember how a mugwump sits on a fence, his mug on one side and the rest of him on the other, ready to fall in any direction he's pushed? Some hidden habits are like that. Starting as harmless cobwebs, if pushed in the wrong direction they fall into the injurious cable category. Here is an example of a mugwump habit and how it can become a cable.

Poor Posture: In the beginning, poor posture may be no more than sagging shoulders that make you look older and less attractive or give you a defeated, hangdog look. That's bad enough. But as it grows worse, poor posture can warp your personality and mental outlook. It can also injure your health. If you don't believe it, try shuffling along with shoulders stooped, stomach protruding, head bowed and chest caved in. Within a matter of minutes, your mood and general outlook can change from cheerfulness and confidence to a state of depression that matches your "I-give-up" slump.

When your body is continually forced out of balance by poor posture, other organs become crowded so they are unable to function as they should without abnormal strain. Since your muscles are constantly in a state of contraction, prolonged sitting, standing and walking out of balance put an excessive burden on them. The result is fatigue, tense nerves, muscular aches and pains. Other mental and physical discomforts caused by poor posture contribute to so-called nervous stomach. Poor posture can also slow down the thinking process. This is due to the decreased intake of oxygen caused by slumped shoulders, caved-in chest and crowded lung capacity.

To overcome bad habits of long standing takes both physical stamina to make the effort and mental health to provide the will power and determination. Whether or not you have them depends upon two other habits—those of good and bad nutrition. Poor nutritional habits are so widespread and their consequences so serious that I have no choice except to list them among the other dangerous habits.

Cable Habits

Poor Nutritional Habits: As a reminder of the difference between good and bad nutrition, the following head our list of worst nutritional habits:

Overeating: Habitual overeating of anything is bad. But the most destructive habit is eating too much of the wrong foods, especially those loaded with hard fats and refined carbohydrates (starches and sugars).

Undereating: Skipping meals, particularly breakfast, is a bad nutritional habit to get into. So is eating too few of the protective foods necessary to prevent deficiencies. Although overeating is usually a faster road to self-destruction, shortchanging yourself of the nutrients your body requires paves the way for a slow and painful journey in the same direction.

Since the subject that led into this was posture, let's take up where we left off by examining some of the food elements that are of value in achieving and maintaining good posture.

1. A diet high in protein is essential to strengthen your body and build strong muscles to support you without sagging under the load.

2. Magnesium, calcium and the B vitamins contribute not only to physical health, but to mental and emotional well-being. Two of the B vitamins, niacin and biotin, the "courage" and "mental health," or "morale," vitamins, help provide qualities necessary to sustain the long-range effort to break bad habits and form good ones.

This is not to minimize the value of all the other vitamins and minerals, some of which are more effective in correcting one condition and some another. *But never forget that all of them are essential to overcoming poor nutritional habits and to forming the good ones that will keep you alive and youthful longer.*

Excessive Smoking: What can I say to you about the effects of excessive smoking that you don't already know? If the horrifying incidence of lung cancer in heavy smokers and the written and verbal warnings of doctors and scientists haven't reached you, I doubt that anything I can say will cause you to break this dangerous habit.

But if you insist you can't quit, and with a life in the balance, let's do what we can to save it by using every available means of protection.

One in particular, according to recent scientific experiments, gives promise of being an important factor in preventing lung cancer. The cost is negligible, and it's as easy as taking a vitamin. Because that's exactly what it is—vitamin A.

At the Ninth International Cancer Congress in Tokyo (October, 1966), important experiments in this area were revealed by Dr. Umberto Saffiotti, a pathologist at the University of Chicago Medical School. In laboratory tests with hamsters, Dr. Saffiotti subjected their lungs to benzpyrene, one of the chief cancer-causing chemicals in cigarettes. Hamsters were chosen for the experiments because they are animals that normally never contract lung cancer. Yet nearly 100 percent of those that were exposed developed the disease.

Then, taking a similar group of hamsters, he administered large doses of vitamin A while exposing them to the same chemicals that had caused lung cancer in the first group. Vitamin A is known to influence the health and functioning of the bronchial lining. Dr. Saffiotti expected to see some change in the rate and manner of tumor development. But the results far surpassed his expectation! *The experiments with the second group of hamsters revealed that vitamin A apparently works to halt or reverse the cancerous growths and to render almost all of the animals who had taken it immune to the disease.*

But scientists are conservative in their estimate of work in progress. Dr. Saffiotti is no exception. His findings, he says, are not yet conclusive, although he admits that they might "lead to results of practical significance for the prevention of lung cancer."

Yet in spite of my great respect for researchers, if I were a smoker and couldn't quit—as many of you say you can't—I wouldn't wait for the final experiments to be in. If I did, it might be too late for *me*. At present, besides eating meals high in protein, vitamins, minerals and enzymes, along with other food supplements, I take 25,000 international units of vitamin A each morning. If I were a heavy smoker I would raise the daily total to 75,000 units, taking one after each meal for better absorption.

Not only is the incidence of death from lung cancer much higher among cigarette smokers, but cancer of the mouth and death from strokes, emphysema, heart attacks and cirrhosis of the liver are up to seven times higher in heavy smokers in the forty-five to sixty age group than in nonsmokers of the same age.

Researchers at Mayo Clinic have found that, on the average, smokers are struck down by coronary thrombosis ten years earlier than nonsmokers. And heavy smoking is believed to be largely responsible for the increasing number of coronaries occurring among women during recent years.

Smokers have 65 percent higher incidence of colds than nonsmokers, 76 percent higher incidence of nervousness, 167 percent higher incidence of nose and throat irritation, 300 percent higher incidence of cough. Smoking destroys vitamin C, the vitamin known to be valuable in preventing many of these conditions and which aids in keeping the tissues, including the lung tissue, healthy.

Just one cigarette will destroy the amount of vitamin C in an orange, which is often the only adequate source of this vitamin in the average diet. If I were a smoker, I would add from 750 to 1,000 milligrams of extra vitamin C to my daily diet, depending on how much I smoked.

Vitamin C is also valuable in preventing or controlling chemical poisoning. It has been used to correct the toxic effects of benzene, lead, bromide, arsenic and other substances with which industrial workers frequently come in contact. Although it has not yet been tried to counteract the effects of poisonous chemicals in cigarettes, its known detoxifying power is another sound reason for every smoker to make sure he gets *more* than enough vitamin C every day of his life. There is no danger of taking too much.

And, finally, if I were a smoker, I would never neglect my daily supplements of vitamin A. I would always keep in mind that it was successful in halting or arresting tumorous growths in the hamsters exposed to cancer-causing chemicals. When something as harmless and beneficial as a vitamin has even the slightest possibility of preventing or arresting a dread disease, I would take advantage of whatever hope it held and say to myself and others, *"What can we lose? Let's try it now—and prove it later!"*

Excessive Drinking: Now and then I remind myself that I am *not* a reformer. And yet, in a way, I must admit that I am. Most of my life has been spent trying to get the eating public—which includes everybody—to improve their nutritional way of life, and that usually means reforming it. So I'm not out to *reform* the heavy drinker, who probably intends to go on drinking just as long as he feels like it. My purpose is to give him some nutritional help that he desperately needs—which can also lessen his desire to drink.

It's an accepted fact that excessive drinking causes serious nutritional problems. Alcohol is known to be a notorious B vitamin robber, causing a B complex deficiency that often shows up in disastrous physical and mental symptoms. It depletes the body's store of other vitamins and minerals, as well.

At the University of California at Los Angeles, Dr. Robert N. Baker reported a study of alcoholics that showed neurological symptoms thought to be caused by heavy drinking were found to result from another cause—the vitamin deficiency it induced! Some of the symptoms resulting from that deficiency are: delirium tremens, convulsions, neuritis, disorders of eye movement, incoordination of gait and impaired memory.

A destruction of certain brain tissue is common among alcoholics. It may begin with some of the symptoms above, including uncoordinated walk, paralysis of the eye muscles and clouding of the consciousness, ending in coma.

A strange type of brain disorder prevalent among heavy drinkers is believed to be caused by a vitamin deficiency. Called *Korsakoff's psychosis,* it may be roughly translated as "psychological liar." The victim is highly suggestible to any wild idea and is completely without judgment concerning it. He is a habitual tellers of fantastic tall tales who imagines his stories to be true. Other changes of the brain, including hemorrhages, often found throughout the brain tissue of chronic alcoholics, have been related to deficiencies of both vitamin C and B complex.

Also caused by a lack of B vitamins is a frequent complication of chronic alcoholism, *polyneuritis,* which is characterized by changes or destruction in the peripheral nerves of the body. A B-Complex supplement, liver, brewer's yeast and other nutritional supplements added to the heavy drinker's diet would prevent this and other painful conditions that are the result of the nutritional deficiencies caused by excessive use of alcohol.

Cirrhosis of the liver, long considered a drunkard's disease, is basically a nutritional problem, brought on by an inadequate diet. Listed by the Metropolitan Life Insurance Company as the fifth leading cause of death among Americans between the ages of forty-five and sixty-four, cirrhosis is most prevalent in persons whose diets are deficient in protein and B vitamins. That, of course, includes the heavy drinker. But the disease occurs just as often in nondrinkers who are victims of the same nutritional deficiencies as the alcoholic.

An effective treatment for the disease was first introduced by Dr. Lester M. Morrison, a prominent California physician, and later used extensively by physicians in all parts of the world. This highly successful treatment is based on high-protein meals combined with vitamin and other nutritional supplements, with additional injections of liver and vitamins. A healthy liver is your best defense against many of the diseases that make you age faster and die younger.

Alcoholism—a Nutritional Disease?

We know that the alcoholic is an accomplice to his own vitamin and mineral robbery. By his excessive drinking and his poor and irregular eating habits, he leaves his body vulnerable to disease. But here is a fact that is not as well known as it should be: *In a surprising number of cases alcoholism itself is a nutritional disease!* (This is not discounting the psychological problems of the alcoholic, many of which are decreased or cured under an improved diet and vitamin and mineral therapy.)

Dr. Roger J. Williams of the University of Texas spent years of research and made countless clinical tests on both animals and humans to prove this theory. His findings have been published in his own book, *Nutrition and Alcoholism,* and in the *Journal of Clinical Nutrition* under the title "Alcoholism As a Nutritional Problem." Here are some of the facts that his experiments revealed:

1. The alcoholic has a higher-than-average requirement for certain food elements, perhaps due to heredity, which causes him to crave something without knowing what it is. He turns to drink to satisfy his unidentified craving. This increases both the

deficiency and his craving, which is now fixed on liquor, and starts a vicious cycle known as "the man takes a drink, the drink takes a drink, then the drink takes the man."

2. The heavy drinker needs an abundance of high-grade protein, never less than seventy grams a day. He should avoid the "empty calories" of refined carbohydrates.

3. A lack of B vitamins proved to be an undeniable factor in the overpowering craving for liquor. Even those taking the occasional social drink should remember that alcohol, like other carbohydrates, needs B vitamins for its metabolism and will rob the body of its store to meet this demand. Deficiencies result unless the supply is continually replenished with B-rich foods and supplements. When alcoholics were given an improved, high-protein diet plus large amounts of B complex the urge to drink was decreased or completely overcome!

If there is a heavy drinker among your friends or in your family, magnesium (as dolomite) added to the high-protein diet and B complex supplements in Dr. Williams' proven plan are invaluable in his rehabilitation. Building up his physical and mental health by correcting the lack that caused his craving will help him overcome his dependence on liquor, loosen the cable bonds of the habit, and finally, enable him to break it completely.

It is important to counteract *immediately* all the habits that contribute to aging, because the longer they persist, the more damage they do and the harder they are to break. Some affect appearance only, making the offender look older than his years; others, such as smoking and excessive drinking, are more serious abuses, because they have a debilitating effect on general health.

I have stressed that in preventing and reversing the undesirable patterns of both kinds of habits, one of the most important elements is proper diet. In addition to good nutrition, and in order to insure healthy circulation and muscle strength, the body also needs constant exercise. When a program of sound nutrition and daily exercise are combined, the body functions at a level of maximum efficiency.

12

Stay Active—or Atrophy!

"The tremendous aptitude for inactivity among Americans might end in a human erosion that could strip the nation of its strength within the next generation." The speaker was Dr. Shane McCarthy, executive director of President Eisenhower's Council on Youth Fitness; the time was December, 1956.

The happenings between then and now have given a sense of prophecy to his words. At the time, he said that his own sons, like other youths, "could hardly wait until they were old enough to give up walking and sit behind the wheel of a car." Today, more and more experts on physical fitness are expressing concern over the "human erosion" taking place in this generation.

"It will come as a shock to the sedentary American male that his body is middle-aged by the time he is 26," says Dr. Thomas Cureton, director of the Physical Fitness Research Laboratory at the University of Illinois. Dr. Cureton gives another jolt to young men when he says, "We define middle age as the 26-to-65 year span during which there is a steady loss of physical abilities." The loss shows up first in a decrease in leg, arm and shoulder strength, then in speed and flexibility. But notice that in Dr. Cureton's first statement he was referring to the *sedentary* male.

When inertia replaces activity in either body or mind, the wasting effects of atrophy begin. (Mental inertia and how to cope with it are taken up in Chapter 18.) The inactive body slows down and loses strength. It gets soft and flabby. Overweight presents a serious threat to health. Unused muscles lose tone. The heart stroke weakens.

The result is a man—or woman—who feels too old, tired and run-down to make the physical effort necessary to prevent or correct these and other symptoms of premature aging. Chronic complaints are far more prevalent in persons who are inactive than they are in active individuals.

In his studies at the University of Michigan, Dr. John C. Tappan found a much higher incidence of fatigue, diabetes, digestive troubles and nervous and cardiovascular disorders in sedentary professors than in those who were active. Another expert who deplores the fact that most Americans become physically inactive by their mid-twenties is Dr. Louis F. Bishop of New York University. Though around this age many young adults become "too busy to exercise," says Dr. Bishop, "in the next two decades of their lives they probably need it even more than do their children."

But it isn't only in America that cars, push buttons and gadget-crammed homes and offices are causing our joints to stiffen while muscles weaken and atrophy from lack of use. Last year I was in Melbourne, Australia, on one of my lecture tours. After an early dinner with friends, my host, Rex Hughes, insisted on driving me to the lecture.

"Why not walk?" I asked.

"Walk?" Rex looked at me as though he never heard the word. "Do you know how far it is? My legs wouldn't make it!"

In appearance, Rex was broad-shouldered and rugged, as are a good many Australians. He was, I knew, at least thirty years my junior. Yet his muscles were as weak and his joints as stiff as those of a feeble old man who hadn't used them for years.

We slowed down as we drove past a midtown Melbourne park and saw schoolgirls playing night basketball, running and leaping with the grace of ballerinas and the vigor of rugby players. I was reminded of a New York sportswriter who once described Australia as "a land entirely surrounded by water and inundated by athletes." "It's a country that has produced champions in such diverse sports as tennis, cricket, billiards, auto racing, sailing, swimming, sculling and running," I thought as we rode past. Then, as though he had been reading my mind, Rex said, "I used to be a pretty good athlete myself. Did a lot of swimming and surfing, played tennis, and was a marathon walker."

"Why did you give them up?" I asked.

"Too busy. Haven't had time for sports since college. And I quit walking when I bought my first car. Riding saves my time —and my legs."

"The only way you can save your legs is by using them," I told him. "And you may save your heart at the same time."

Before I left Australia, I gave Rex six time-saving but effective exercises (see page 115) and advised him to get in some walking every day, even if he had to park his car several blocks from his office. But he didn't start reconditioning himself until a light heart attack warned him that inactivity was a threat to his life.

Sedentary habits threaten the health of Britons, too, according to health officer Dr. N. E. Chadwick of Hove, England. *"Today's killer is inactivity!"* he says. (My italics) He is convinced that inactivity is responsible for the rapid rise in illness and early death, especially among men. He thinks that the stresses and insecurities of modern living have been accused when they are not to blame, since "some form of insecurity has been present with every generation." There is no easy answer to the problems facing us. But if we lose the physical, mental and moral stamina required to make the effort, they will never be solved, either on a personal or national level.

Dr. Edward Bortz, a former president of the American Medical Association, says that a loss of stamina and premature old age can be caused by muscles wasting away through disuse.

The body contains two different sets of muscles: the voluntary and involuntary. The involuntary muscles work automatically, so we don't have to worry about them. What we want to do is condition the voluntary muscles and prevent their atrophy.

Our body has 700 voluntary muscles, large and small. We use them when we stand, walk, jog, run, push, pull, reach, stretch, wiggle, flex, lift, bend, stoop, turn, twist or carry on almost any physical activity—even sitting. (But you won't strengthen any muscles just by sitting—unless you do a few isometric exercises at the same time.) The above list of body movements should give you a clue to the necessary types of exercise. "Every muscle and joint that has the power to wiggle," says Dr. Howard Ross of the Michigan State Medical Society, "must be made to wiggle more."

A brain surgeon advises the same practices, not only to improve circulation and ease the heart's job of pumping blood to the brain, but to prevent the deterioration of other faculties. "Wiggle your toes frequently," says Dr. Bruce V. Kvernland of Portland, Oregon, "and keep moving your arms and legs around if you want to protect your mental faculties, sight and hearing from deteriorating with age."

Both men and women can put a little more reaching, stretching and bending into everyday movements. There are many ways of putting "hidden exercises" into routine activities to help maintain firm muscles and flexible bodies.

The Royal Canadian Air Force exercise booklets suggest balancing on one foot while you put on your shoes and socks. If you need a wider area to balance on, it's right behind you. Try sitting on the floor, raising both legs in the air and balancing on your buttocks while you pull on your socks or nylons. If done correctly, your body will form a *V* shape in midair—and you can feel your leg, back and abdominal muscles getting a workout.

One woman I know polishes her floors and reduces her hips at the same time. She puts on an old pair of jeans and spreads a large polishing cloth on the floor. Then she sits on the cloth and scoots around the floor, rocking from side to side to give her excess fat a thumping as she polishes.

"I know it looks undignified," she says, "but it's practical!"

If you want less conspicuous ways of firming and toning muscles, you might work some of the following into your daily routine.

Isometric Exercises

Isometric exercises, tensing one set of muscles against another or against an immovable object, can be done almost anywhere, to tone, firm and strengthen the muscles. There is nothing new about these exercises, except their current widespread popularity. For years physiotherapists have used isometrics to prevent the atrophy of muscles in arms or legs encased in plaster. The U.S. Marines have isometric exercises designed for their office personnel and others in sedentary occupations. In just one minute of isometrics a day as they sat in the office, it took only twenty weeks for desk-bound Marines to double the strength of the muscles they exercised!

The businessman and woman can do partial push-ups as they rise from the desk by bracing their palms against it and pushing the body to a standing position. The housewife can do the same as she gets up from the kitchen table. Or if she hasn't had time to sit, she can do it by leaning at a forward angle against the kitchen sink and pushing herself erect.

Although isometrics can't take the place of exercises that carry oxygen to the blood and stimulate the circulation, nearly everyone can benefit from them. The exception is the person with circulatory or respiratory disorders, who should get professional advice before attempting any except the mildest isometric contractions. Because of a reflex action beyond voluntary control, strong contractions can arrest his blood circulation.

Remember to hold the tension in each exercise for at least six seconds—and don't forget to breathe freely as you do them.

Waist and Abdomen

This is one of the best-known and most popular isometrics. Sometimes called the "stomach lift," it's widely used by motion picture stars and other men and women in public life to whittle the waistline and flatten the abdomen. It can be done anywhere —sitting, standing or lying down. Simply tighten the abdominal muscles, contracting them as hard as you can—try to feel your stomach being pulled back to meet your backbone—and hold for six seconds, or until the muscles quiver from tension.

Waist, Abdomen and Legs

This one is done on the floor. Sit with legs apart, back straight and weight partially supported on arms. Contract stomach muscles with enough force to lift legs off floor. Keep leg muscles tensed, hold for a count of six. Don't get up yet! Stay on the floor for the next one.

Legs, Abdomen, Chest and Arms

If you've ever watched a magician's levitation trick, you can visualize this exercise. Lie flat on your back and try to raise yourself horizontally off the floor by contracting all your muscles. You obviously cannot raise yourself in this way, but it's fine for your muscles to *think* they can—and make the attempt.

Legs, Waist, Abdomen, Arms (and Other Assorted Muscles)

This one is done standing, anywhere, any time. It takes a little imagination, too. Brace your feet hard against the floor—harder—as though you're trying to dig them into it. Before six seconds are up, you'll feel the contraction in nearly every muscle in your body.

Arms, Legs and Abdomen

Sit upright in a chair with your hands resting on your knees. Then press your hands down as hard as you can for six seconds, while trying to lift your knees.

Abdomen, Arms, Legs and Thighs

Sit well back on a chair, hold your legs straight out and place the palms of your hands above your kneecaps. Press downward with your arms and upward with your legs, against strong resistence.

Ankle Flex

In a sitting or standing position, attempt to flex the foot upward from the ankle joint. Resistence can be exerted by the hands or some other object. This exercise strengthens front muscles of the lower legs.

Chest and Arms

This one firms and strengthens arms and is a chest developer for men and bosom firmer for women. Bend arms in front of chest, interlock fingers and hold palms flat together. Press hard and hold until the pectoral muscles quiver with tension.

Chest and Arms—Variation in Two Parts

1. Double your fists and at the same time pull your arms back and up, trying to touch the elbow. Hold for ten counts.
2. Clasp hands in front of you at waist level; contract arm and chest muscles, pushing palms together.

Arms and Neck

Place the palm of the left hand against the left side of the head. Press with the head against the hand. Repeat on the right-hand side, front and back of the head. This strengthens weak neck muscles.

Shoulder, Chest and Arms (Standing)

Stand in the center of a doorway, feet comfortably spread. Place the hands against the sides of the doorway so that they are at shoulder height. That means the arms will be bent and palms will be touching the sides of the doorjamb. Press against the sides—hard.

Shoulder, Chest and Arms (Sitting)

While seated, grasp the arms of your chair firmly, lift hard for six seconds, as though you were trying to raise them up to your shoulders. Or, from the same position, press down on the chair arms just as hard as you can for six seconds.

Forearms, Chest and Upper Arms

Use the "isometric squeeze." Hold your hands tightly together, palms facing, then press them against each other for six seconds. To reverse this, fold your hands tightly together, then try to pull them apart for six full seconds.

Upper Arms and Back

Stand in a doorjamb, taking a wide-leg stance, with back straight. Press both palms against jamb, first at hip level, then as high as you can reach. In each position push with maximum force while counting slowly to ten. Keep spine straight.

Upper Back and Arms

Yes, these are similar, but different back muscles are used in varying degrees, as you'll see when you try them. Stand about twelve to eighteen inches away from a wall, back facing the wall. With the arms alongside of the body, place the palms against the wall. Keeping the arms straight, exert a pressure against the wall, as though attempting to push it down.

Forearm and Grip

You can do this from either a sitting or standing position. Hold your arms out loosely, with your fingers outstretched; then stretch your fingers as far apart as you can, as though you were trying to tear your hands apart. For the reverse of this, form a fist with each hand and then squeeze your fingers together hard.

What Isometrics Will Not *Do*

Isometric exercises should be used in *addition* to other exercises, not as a substitute for them. They can't take the place of what the Air Force conditioning program calls aerobic exercises. Aerobics are the exercises that cover a range of body movements that are vigorous enough to stimulate the circulatory system, benefit the blood system, flush the tissues with oxygen, reinvigorate the muscle-nourishing capillaries and aid in preventing the accumulation of fat deposits in the arteries. Isometrics will not perform any of these vital functions.

The exercises that will, and which can prolong your life and perhaps prevent a heart attack, are given later in the chapter. But before we get to those, here are some of the specialized exercises I promised you.

Sexercises

It was Bonnie Prudden who coined the term "sexercises," referring to those exercises that, in addition to promoting general fitness, were of value in sexual relations. She initiated the routine of firming and strengthening the muscles and organs used in the following sexercises, and called them first aid for ailing marriages. The fact is, however, that it takes a *combination* of sound nutrition and physical activity to give both men and women the health and vigor necessary for satisfactory marriage relations.

Mrs. Prudden acknowledges that "the muscles one needs for sex are also essential for many sports." So if you've kept yourself in good physical condition by one or more daily sports or by some regular aerobic exercises, you may not need sexercises. But if your back, thighs, legs and hips are weak and stiff, and your muscles—especially the very important gluteal and abdominal muscles—are limp and lax from inactivity, sexercises will improve them.

Kinesiology, the science of muscular movement, reveals that the *gluteus maximus,* the big muscle on the back of the hips, is strengthened most effectively either by tensing, pushing, thrusting or kicking against the resistance of opposing muscles or by exercises that raise the legs past a forty-five-degree angle. You'll see how often isometrics are combined with these exercises, which is one of the reasons we had them first. I wanted you to be familiar with the tensing and resisting principles before we started sexercises.

Gluteal and Abdominal Squeeze

Basically, this consists of pulling your back in toward your front. Practice it first lying down; later it can be done, like the stomach lift, sitting up, standing and almost anywhere. Lie on your stomach, head resting on curved arms or a pillow. Tighten your gluteal muscles by pinching your buttocks together as hard as you can, pulling in your abdominal muscles at the same time (as in the stomach lift, only make the two simultaneous). Hold for six seconds, or approximately to the count of ten, then relax completely before the next one. Start with three and work up to at least ten repetitions—twice a day, if you can.

Gluteal, Abdominal and Back Stretch

Stay on your stomach for this one, only stretch your arms up to rest vertically on the floor above your head. Tense buttocks, back and shoulder muscles with enough force to lift the legs and upper torso slightly off the floor, with toes and arms still on the floor. Hold for a slow count of ten. Repeat twice to start, gradually working up to eight or ten.

Abdominal and Back Flex

While you're on your stomach, you might as well try balancing on it with this one. Put hands behind neck, keeping legs rigid. Tense the lower back muscles and raise head, chest and feet as high as you can, tensing your midsection to support the part of you in midair. Count to five and relax.

And right here is a good place to say that except in some instances, you can decide for yourself how many repetitions your muscles will stand without groaning. Let moderation be the key word at first, in any case. We want to strengthen your muscles, not make them ache. Then work up to what seems to be the best number of repetitions for you, which will probably average around ten. If more are needed in some exercises, I'll tell you.

Knee Lift and Backward Stretch

This improves muscle strength and flexibility (as all the sexercises do). It also aids circulation and helps relieve stiffness and tension in back, neck and shoulder muscles. Get down on your hands and knees. Bend right leg and lift knee up to touch your chest. Stretch leg behind you. Raise it as high as you can, back arched and gluteals tensed. (Remember that a forty-five-degree-or-more angle strengthens them.) Repeat five times with right leg, the same with the left. Gradually work up to ten repetitions with each leg.

Leg, Abdominal and Thigh Flex

Lie on your back, legs together, hands behind your head. Raise legs until they're about eighteen inches from the floor, then stretch them apart as far as you can. Hold until you feel the muscles quiver. Then, with legs still elevated, bring them together again and lower slowly to the floor.

Semisplit and Slide

Like the preceding exercise, this one also develops strength and flexibility in the thigh adductors. Stand with feet a few inches apart. Slowly slide feet farther apart, as though you were going to the floor in a dancer's split—only stop halfway or when you feel a definite stretch in your crotch. Still keeping legs straight, slide them together again by using a heel-toe foot movement.

Lying-Down Knee Lift and Thigh Flex

Lie on back, with arms stretched on the floor at shoulder level, palms down. Draw knees up to chest, keeping toes pointed and hips on the floor. Without moving head, arms or shoulders, rotate knees and thighs to the left and touch your left knee to the floor. Repeat on the right side with right knee.

Bottoms Up

This strengthens the gluteal and back muscles, but if you have a back that gives you trouble, better wait until you've limbered up before trying it. Lie on stomach, head cushioned on arms. Keeping chest firmly on the floor, let knees and chest support you. Raise buttocks high in the air until body resembles an upside-down *V*. Tighten gluteals and hold for a count of four, then relax. Six repetitions should be plenty.

Hip Swing and Thrust

Stand with knees straight and feet slightly apart. Tighten the gluteals, abdominals, thigh muscles and knees. Then, without turning or twisting the body, with a firm thrust, swing the hips as far to the right as possible. Keep muscles tightened and swing to the left. This conditions the pelvic area to move by itself as a compact unit, without involving other movements of the body. Alternate hips for a total of twelve swings (six for each side).

For Women Only

Before we get to the tenth and final sexercise, the pelvic tilt, which is probably the most important of all, I want to tell you about a technique that can benefit all women. It's easy to do once you've mastered it, and it can be practiced standing, sitting or lying down.

A levator is a muscle that serves to raise some part of the body, and there is one lying along the floor of the pelvis. By combining an alternate tensing and relaxing of the levator, the gluteals and the abdominals, the inner muscles can be firmed and tightened. You already know how to tense and relax the gluteals and abdominals. But to perfect the same technique with the levator, it may help you to remember how, as a child, you hated to interrupt play for a call to dinner—or any other call. Think, for example, of the inner muscles you involuntarily tightened so you could postpone a trip to the bathroom. Think hard—and tighten hard!—until the levator will respond to your conscious command.

The exercise itself is easy: Simply tighten the levator, the gluteals and abdominals, hold a second, then relax completely. Start with 20 a day and work up to 80 or 100 for best results. They can be done at intervals, whenever you think of it, in sets of 20 or 30 at a time. Regular practice will improve the firmness, flexibility and control of the inner muscles and the overall pelvic region.

The Pelvic Tilt

The pelvic tilt, or thrust, is one of the basic exercises recommended by experts on the subject. You may have learned it in gym class at school, and forgotten about it unless you had occasion to use it later to perfect your form in tennis, skiing or other sport. Watch a skier coming down a curved slope, and you can see how essential the forward, backward and sideways movement of the pelvis is to him. Practice his movements for the standing pelvic tilt. Don't forget to tighten the abdomen and buttocks (and women the levator) at the same time. And to strengthen some of the little-used inner muscles, combine the standing pelvic tilt and the hip swing and thrust.

Pelvic tilt prone: Lying on stomach, arch back slightly, tighten and raise buttocks, pull pelvis up and forward, hold briefly then relax. Start with four repetitions, working up to eight or ten.

Pelvic tilt sitting: Sit in a straight chair and arch body forward, with head toward knees. Tuck buttocks under and tighten other muscles. Then with a backward rolling motion, tilt pelvis upward, support weight with feet on the floor and hands on the side of the chair, and raise rigid body an inch or so in the air. This can also be done sitting on the floor, but until your arm muscles have strengthened, raising the body is done more easily with hands braced on a chair.

There are many variations of the pelvic tilt, but all of them include the muscle tightening, the tucking under, tilting up, and the forward, backward and sometimes sideways movements in varying degrees, whether they are done lying down, sitting, standing, bending over or walking. Many girls use it automatically in walking, some more than others.

Pelvic tilt bending over: The best description I can give you of this one is to tell you how as a boy, I used to stand outside the fence around the baseball park, bent over, hands on my knees, peeking at the game through a knothole in the fence. Now, imagine you're that little boy and the manager came up behind you and smacked you on the bottom. The fence blocks your getaway, so your involuntary reaction would be to tighten your buttocks to ward off the blow and give a quick forward thrust to your pelvis to lunge out of danger. Well, that's the way it's done. And it should give you an idea of how you can develop many of your own variations of the pelvic tilt.

Done consistently, sexercises will amply reward both men and women. For women, the special fringe benefits are these: They firm and strengthen lax interior muscles, contribute to the health of the overall pelvic region, help prevent backache and swayback, and are an excellent conditioner after childbirth. They will give to both sexes stronger, more flexible muscles, trim, firm hips and derriere, a flat abdomen, and the increased resilience, strength of body and muscular control that add up to a more satisfactory sex life.

Six Time-Saver Conditioners

In addition to long, brisk walks, these are the conditioners that I personally use and have recommended to many men and women who think they are too busy to exercise. Most of you will recognize these exercises. Some of you may have tried a few occasionally. But no matter how good the exercise is, doing it *occasionally* won't keep you fit. "Exercise for general fitness does not have to be extremely vigorous," says New York University's Dr. Roscoe Brown. "It is more important that it be regular."

You can do these six exercises in a little more or less than five minutes a day, depending on how fast you do them and the time you spend relaxing between sets.

1. *The Stretcher*

Stand with the feet apart and hands clasped loosely in front of you. Relax the body and drop it downward from the waist, head dangling toward the floor. Then, using the hips as a pivot, with hands still clasped but arms extended, sweep the upper body in a wide circle, sideways, upward as high as you can stretch, and backward; then circle down the other side and toward the floor again, touching it with your fingers if you can. Continue circling in an unbroken rhythm, five times clockwise and five counter-clockwise. This is good for limbering up, and it's of special benefit to the hamstring muscles and spine.

2. *Forward and Backward Kick*

Stand with the left hand resting against the wall or a chair back for balance. Swing the right leg forward and up as high as you can, then backward as far as possible. Keep the knee relaxed so it flexes naturally as the leg swings back. As the knee bends on the backward kick, you'll feel the workout in the quadriceps muscles of the thigh. Do six front and back kicks with each leg to start, working up to more as your flexibility increases.

3. *The Knee Hug*

The name of this exercise practically describes it. Better stand against a wall at first for balance. Raise one leg and lift the knee as close to the chest as you can. Then, putting both arms around it, draw it close to the body and hold it against the chest. Ten knee hugs for each leg should be about right.

Variations: You can double up on this one by drawing both

knees to the chest at the same time as you're sitting watching TV or when you're lying flat on your back in bed.

4. Partial Sit-Up

Lie on back, with arms at your side and feet slightly apart. Slowly raise head and shoulders from the floor high enough to see the length of your feet and to feel the pull in abdominal muscles and shoulders. Hold long enough to count your toes; then lower yourself slowly to the floor.

5. Partial Push-Up

You had one version of this in isometric exercises, but to be sure you'll include it in your time-saver conditioners, here's another way of doing it, just as simple but a little more strenuous.

Stand well back from a windowsill, arms straight out and hands on the sill to support your forward-leaning body. Lower yourself on arms until chin touches the sill, then slowly straighten arms to push body up to a standing position. Representative Fred Schwengel of Iowa, a former physical education teacher, does 600 full push-ups a day, and alternates them with other exercises. But unless your condition is as good as his, you'd better start with 6. And just partial push-ups, at that. If you want to be sure of privacy, you can do them against the side of the bathtub, instead of at the window. Just be sure to cover it with a Turkish towel so your hands won't slip.

6. Running in Place

Sometimes called treadmill running or indoor jogging, this is the most important of the indoor exercises, and you'll hear more of its benefits in the next chapter. Vigorous use of the leg muscles aids the body's circulatory system and, as Dr. Paul Dudley White explains it, "When the leg muscles contract, they squeeze the veins (which have valves) and actually pump blood up toward the heart. This allows the heart to receive more blood."

You do it exactly the same way you'd jog outside, only you stay in one place. Start with a brisk marking-time movement to get into it if you like, lifting the knees and raising the feet about two inches off the floor. Then quicken steps to a running or jogging pace, with elbows loosely bent and arms swinging back and forth, as you've seen runners or other athletes in training do.

Begin with about a minute, or approximately a count of 100, then work up to two, three, four and five minutes, or more as you can. Or you can fit several sessions of one minute each into a busy day during convenient intervals. For a more vigorous workout when time is limited, go a little faster and raise knees higher. If your heart starts racing and you get short of breath, don't worry about it. It's a normal reaction. One of the benefits of vigorous exercise is that it forces the heart to pump faster to meet the body's increasing need for more oxygen-rich blood. Dr. Laurence E. Morehouse, professor of physical education at UCLA and a strong advocate of jogging, gives this general rule to go by: "When your heart pounds, it isn't a warning signal. But if your head pounds—stop!"

Bob Bauman, trainer of the St. Louis Cardinals and a member of the physical education staff at St. Louis University, believes that for athletes, executives and everyone "the ideal conditioner is daily running, whether it be on a treadmill (running in place) or running outside." The Cardinals' exercise program includes running, a twisting-and-bending routine, handball for some of the players, and a simple hand exercise for all of them. Bauman has found that reaching the arms high above the head "keeps atrophy from getting to the muscles in the shoulder area. Aids respiration and even helps the heart muscle to stay in shape." His parting words to his players are these: "If you don't do anything else, at least raise your arms above your head twenty times each day." That's easy and beneficial advice that anyone can follow. It's up to you whether you drag around with a middle-aged body by the time you're twenty-six—or stay active and physically fit well into old age.

An active life with adequate exercise helps you keep physically fit. It also makes you sexually more responsive. Turn to the next chapter to see how to maintain—and increase—your sexual vigor.

13

Sexual Vigor After Forty

Why is it that some men and women retain their sexual vigor and sex appeal so much longer than others? There are a number of reasons for it. Some of them are physical. Some are psychological. An early decline of sexual powers may result from a glandular imbalance. A run-down condition, prolonged illness or chronic disease can cause either a temporary or a progressive decline. So can any one of many nutritional deficiencies that throw the body chemistry and endocrine system out of balance. Anxieties, unfulfilled emotional needs, repressed hostilities, an unrelieved fear-stress syndrome and other psychological factors account for a large share of sexual failure among men of all ages.

But whether the cause is physical, psychological, or a combination of both, this chapter will tell you what science has found to be the best methods of preventing the premature loss of your sexual vigor.

The myth that a sudden decline of male potency occurs at middle age should be exploded once and for all! Sexual decline does not occur suddenly or at any predetermined age. Its tempo may decelerate over a period of many years, but so slowly as to be scarcely perceptible—for a man in good physical and emotional health!

Two Duke University scientists, Drs. Gustave Newman and Claude Nichols, gave this 1960 report of their study of men and women ranging in age from sixty to ninety-three:

"Although older persons experience a decline in strength of sexual drive, *given the conditions of reasonably good health, they continue to be sexually active into their seventh, eighth and ninth decades.*" (My italics)

Data collected by Dr. Flanders Dunbar, a noted authority on sex, offers even more encouragement to the beleaguered middle-aged male who may already be gripped by the fear of impotency. In studies of twenty percent of all the men and women one hundred years old or older in America, Dr. Dunbar found that many of the men retained their potency and that some remarried after passing the century mark. When these elders were asked at what age they lost interest in sex, with only one exception, all of them replied in a single word: "Never!" The exception was a recent bridegroom of one hundred and two, who paused to give his wife a hearty kiss before answering. "You've come to the wrong place," he said. "You'll have to ask somebody older than I am!"

Another remarkable case history is of a man one hundred and six years old, reported in a recent psychiatric journal by Dr. Davis B. Schuster of Rochester, New York. Here are the condensed facts of Dr. Schuster's report:

> He noted some decline in libido in his seventies, and at age 106 he still had sexual interests . . . *His physical condition was very good,* showing only a mild degree of anemia and minimal impairment of heart function . . . *He gave the impression of being an alert, vital, and versatile individual with very strong resources whose main anxieties were concerned with a fear of regression and impotency.* (My italics)

"But these men are the exceptions," some of you will probably say. Measured by our present rule of aging, they *are* exceptional. But why? A few key words in the paragraph above give the answer. Keeping in *good physical condition,* staying *alert, vital, versatile* and having *strong resources* helped them retain their sexual vigor until they were one hundred or past and made them the exceptions. Yet any normal man can follow their pattern of aging with exceptional results. *You* can do the same. But instead of thinking of it as a pattern of *aging,* I like to consider it a *"pattern of staying young all your life."*

A number of well-known men who have done just that were the subject of a *Look* magazine article called "In Praise of Older Men." It is interesting to note that the wives of these men never thought of them as old! Here are the tributes two of them paid their noted husbands:

"I have no idea of what it's like to be married to an older man," said Kitty Bradley of her husband, seventy-six-year-old General Omar N. Bradley. "He is the youngest man I know—*vibrant, handsome, virile.*" Mrs. Edward Steichen considers her husband "a great achiever." She is proud of the fact that, as he is nearing ninety, he is not content to be merely one of the world's greatest photographers, but has started a new career as a sculptor.

Dr. Frank Caprio, noted for his research on the sexually adequate male, says that long-term vigor and virility result from a combination of physical and mental health—the quality of being a "whole person." Certainly the examples given so far fit that description.

But there are also less fortunate men who, for a number of reasons, suffer an early decline that could, in most cases, be prevented.

From the middle-aged man to the very old, impotence often results less from physical causes than from the *belief* and the growing *fear* that aging causes loss of virility. These anxieties start a chain reaction. One fear begets another and he begins to feel, look and act old. Unless he can understand his fears and master them, they actually hasten his physical, psychological and sexual decline.

A false belief has made these fears worse—the myth that the male genital system is like a tank that time empties of its contents until nothing is left. The actual truth is this: Impotency is *not* a normal part of life at *any* age for a man in good physical and emotional health. *Nature has set no fixed limitation on sexual capacity.* But when frustration and fear of impotency hamper a man, and he has a few failures, he doesn't stop to realize that there are many reasons for a temporary impotency, and that it needn't be permanent.

Any woman whose husband is going through such a period should give him all the help and encouragement that he needs. Take every opportunity to reassure him of your confidence in his ability as a lover. Never, *never* laugh at his ineffectiveness. Laughter or ridicule at the wrong moment can destroy his self-image and create an emotional block that might cost you his love. Let him know that you understand such temporary lapses, and do your best to convince him that they *are* only temporary.

The two factors largely responsible for maintaining youth and vigor are *an efficient endocrine gland system and a positive protein balance of the body*. These factors are interdependent. If the function of even one gland is impaired, the entire endocrine system is thrown out of balance, the hormonal system loses its equilibrium, and the body goes into what is known as negative protein balance.

Dr. William H. Masters, an eminent gynecologist, pioneer in sexual physiology, and author of *Human Sexual Response,* describes negative protein balance in this way:

"He looks and acts and feels old . . . Deterioration occurs everywhere when an individual stays in negative protein balance—musculature, nerves, brain, blood. His joints stiffen up, his posture ages (when protein balance is lost, bones are unable to retain their calcium) . . . he may develop thin arms and legs but a heavy paunch. He can't understand why he is so tired all the time . . . Any number of signs of mental involution occur . . . *His sex drive diminishes.*" (My italics)

But just as other noted scientists, gerontologists and nutritionists have done, Dr. Masters refutes the common belief that impotence is part of the aging process. "Aging is blamed when it is not the cause," he says. "Certainly it is clear that impotence that develops with age often has to do with poor physical condition and reflects a hormone deficiency . . ."

The body's hormone balance generally reaches its highest level between the ages of twenty to forty. Sometime during the second forty years the glands may begin to slow down. When this results in an uneven production of hormones, it causes an imbalance in the hormonal system, followed by a negative protein balance in the body. These factors, not age, are the conditions Dr. Masters described as being mainly responsible for the diminishing sex drives and other symptoms associated with aging.

The sex glands' production of testosterone (the male hormone, sometimes called androgen) almost always slows down during later years. When a serious deficiency exists, many doctors favor injections of the hormone. Patients are often enthusiastic about this treatment because they expect it to restore their once-youthful sexual vigor. But any man who considers taking it should first have a complete physical examination. If he has ever suffered a serious illness, especially involving the kidneys, heart or liver, or if cancer is suspected, many doctors will advise against the injections. A prominent endocrinologist of New York's Mount Sinai Hospital, Dr. David R. Jacobs, gives this warning:

> Testosterone can be a clinically useful agent in selected cases. However, because of possible adverse side effects, I believe the indiscriminate or routine administration of testosterone should be avoided. Reported side effects include enlargement of the prostate, fluid retention and stimulation of certain cancers already present.

More harmful though usually temporary side effects experienced by many men are an outbreak of pimples, a gain in weight and some nausea.

Do the benefits of testosterone therapy outweigh the danger of its possible adverse side effects? Not in the way and to the extent that most men hope it will, according to another gland specialist, Dr. Herman H. Rubin, who, although he recommends that a deficiency be rectified, adds: "Testosterone stimulates muscle strength and general metabolism. Oddly, this does not appear to be a sex-specific quality."

Dr. Masters has expressed almost the same opinion. He tells of finding "a resurgence of physical strength and mental awareness" in scores of aging men who received therapy. His study in *Human Sexual Response* notes the fact that "androgens (testosterone) and estrogen-androgen combinations" are being used with increasing frequency, not only for the aging male, but for younger men with a sex-hormone imbalance. (Of course, neither male nor female sex hormones should ever be used without expert professional supervision.) But the results of the treatment were not as dramatic as most men had hoped. "There has been some evidence of reawakened sexual interest," the report acknowledged. But the majority of men had hoped for a resurgence of sexual *ability,* not only interest. And not just "some evidence," but a guarantee, though, of course, no guarantee is possible.

Hormone therapy will improve sexual vigor and virility in cases where a sexual decline results solely from a lack of the sex hormone. But this is far from being the only reason for impotency.

Many other factors are almost always involved, including psychological factors. In fact, Dr. Caprio and other authorities list psychological factors as being responsible for about ninety percent of cases of impotency. Here is a list of the most common causes of sexual failure in men:

Major Factors in Male Impotency

1. Psychological. A few of the psychological factors were listed at the beginning of the chapter. It would be impossible to name them all, but here are some that are most often encountered: Fear of failure. Lack of knowledge about sex or faulty attitudes toward it. Self-pity, anger, jealousy or a desire to "get even" with one's mate for some real or imagined reason. Frustration, anxieties and stress.

2. Glandular deficiencies. (See how to keep your glands healthy later in the chapter.)

3. The negative protein balance of the body, already described by Dr. Masters, which follows an imbalance of the hormonal system.

4. Ailments of the prostate gland. (More about this later, too.)
5. Infectious diseases, including venereal disease.
6. Other debilitating diseases.
7. Inflammatory vaginal conditions or vaginal spasms in women, causing pain in the male.
8. Fatigue, of which there are several categories: pathological fatigue, which precedes and follows an illness; emotional fatigue, sometimes a psychological factor, is the hardest to cope with; the easiest to recover from is physical fatigue that results from an excess of either work or play, from too many parties, too little sleep or sports that are too strenuous. It is also the easiest to prevent, since it usually results from causes that are within your control.

When a man is exhausted both physically and mentally, he has neither the desire nor the energy for sex. French actress Jeanne Moreau must have had such men in mind when she said, "Most people don't have the energy for passion, so they give up and go to the movies." Or sit at home and doze in front of the television, she might have added.

9. Drugs and chemicals. Various drugs used for hypertension have been known to cause impotence by blocking certain nerves in the spinal cord. Drugs that depress the central nervous system will cause a loss of potency, ranging from partial to complete. Habitual users of sedatives, tranquilizers and narcotics suffer a loss of virility, and those addicted to large doses of barbiturates and opiates will usually become impotent.

10. Nutritional deficiencies. A balance of foods high in protein, vitamins and minerals is essential in maintaining sexual vigor. A lack of any essential nutrient weakens sexual responses, increases your susceptibility to fatigue, neuroses and various diseases, and makes you an easy target for most of the other factors in impotency.

Sometimes a man will have very little wrong with him except that he has substituted other gratifications for the need to make love. The man so engrossed in his work that he takes his briefcase to bed with him instead of his wife obviously makes a cold bed partner. The overweight man who has substituted an overindulgence in rich food for the need to love and be loved is eating his way into loss of health and early impotence. Dr. George Belham, famous for his *Virility Diet,* claims that obesity is one of the worst enemies of virility. "Sex is not given a starter's chance," he says, "when the stomach is bloated with starch and fat."

Dr. Belham also feels that wives are often guilty of sexual sabotage by undermining a man's potency. They do it by nagging, by excessive emotional and material demands, by an attitude of bedroom boredom, coldness, or the desire to punish a husband. The overly aggressive and demanding wife can do it by making a man feel like an underachiever. And the one who constantly finds fault with her husband and belittles him can destroy his self-confidence along with his potency. Untidy personal habits can also kill sexual response in both men and women.

Often both sexes are to blame for allowing their marriage to settle into a dull, unvarying routine, and letting themselves drift into the state of "humdrum you and monotonous me!"

A satisfying and stimulating relationship with a warm, understanding woman who can meet his particular needs will help a man prolong his sexual vigor. A woman must also have an understanding mate, one who is responsive to her individual needs. And women, like men, have certain very specific requirements and problems related to sex and aging.

Age, Sex and Women

Most women in good health—even those in their seventies and eighties—undergo very little loss in sexual desire due to aging, according to the Kinsey studies and other comprehensive reports. When the ovaries cease to function after the menopause or if they have been removed, one of the compensating factors is a greater production of gonadotropin in women.

Frigidity in women does not result from aging. In women whose health is normal, frigidity is predominantly psychological, not physical. Some women who have always been cold simply stop trying to hide it as they grow older. By the time they reach middle age, they may feel they have a good excuse. They can blame it on the menopause, or they can say, "We're getting too old for that!"

That age has almost nothing to do with it is substantiated by the fact that the female sex hormones play a very minor part in sexual desire. In many cases, women who are past the menopause or those who have had their ovaries removed show a decided increase in desire. One reason for that is the fact that fear can cause inhibitions—and they no longer have to fear an unwanted pregnancy. Consequently, a woman's sexual response may increase, rather than diminish, as she grows older.

In some older women, the muscular support of the pelvis becomes weakened; the pelvic structures lose their firmness; and the womb and bladder tend to drop. (See "Sexercises" in the previous chapter to help keep muscular support firm.) The condition of "dropped uterus" is known technically as *procidentia.* The weakening of the bladder wall is called *cystocele.* These problems, associated with weakness of the vaginal walls, can cause sexual relations to be less satisfactory. The condition can be easily corrected.

Now do you see why you girls—and grandmothers!—were not included in all the discussions of sexual vigor after forty? Most of you don't need it! Your physical and emotional problems of sex as you grow older are different from those of men. And by comparison, yours are relatively minor.

About the Menopause

The menopause is a problem for some women, though, fortunately, not for all. Women who have the most trouble are those whose physical and emotional health is below normal to start with. Also those whose mental outlook is clouded by fear, anxieties and old superstitions. Other women who have a particularly difficult time are those whose adrenal glands are exhausted.

A diet deficient in the nutrients essential to physical and emotional health can cause difficulties at any time, but especially during this period involving what psychologists call a crisis in identity. Of special importance during the menopause and as a preventive measure in the years preceding it are foods rich in protein, vitamins A, B complex (particularly pantothenic acid), C, D, E, and the minerals calcium and magnesium.

The menopause increases the need for vitamin E from ten to fifty times above that of normal. Women suffering from night sweats and hot flashes can often find relief by taking 100 to 500 units daily of the alpha tocopherol form of vitamin E. The B vitamins, the minerals magnesium and calcium, and lecithin help relax tense nerves and build up nerve stability. Lecithin has been called food for the nerves, food for the brain, food for the sex glands, and the greatest nutritional discovery in the past fifty years. Lecithin is found in almost every cell and organ in the body. Adding this remarkable food substance to your diet can, among other benefits, strengthen your nerves and your general health and improve your physical, mental and sexual vigor.

A diet high in protein and other essential nutrients, supplemented with extra amounts of lecithin, calcium, magnesium, and vitamins A, B, C, D and E, will aid your body, nerves and glands in weathering the strains of readjustment during the menopause. And it will help keep you looking and feeling younger in the years ahead.

For both sexes, an abundance of sex hormones, produced and secreted in the ovaries by women and by the testicles in men, depends upon the condition of the glands that produce them. When their production is seriously impaired, the glands must be restored to health, or supplementary measures may be indicated. Yet you have seen that healthy sex glands are not wholly responsible for whether sex lasts a lifetime—or withers prematurely. For sexual desire and ability to endure, you need the health and balance of your mind and body.

It's true that when we see men and women with long-lasting sex appeal and vigor, we may rightly assume that their sex glands are in excellent condition. But there is another gland that is vitally involved in maintaining sexual vigor. The pituitary, or "boss," gland, literally hangs in the back of the skull, suspended on a sort of stalk at the base of the brain. Among its many important functions, it produces the gonadotropic hormone that controls the sex glands. The gonadotropic hormone gives orders to the gonads (the male and female sex glands, the testicles in men and the ovaries in women), which produce the sex hormones, testosterone and estrogen. But it isn't your sex hormones that create the first stirring of sexual interest that you feel. The gonadotropic hormones send the message that starts it all.

As I mentioned earlier, the failure of one gland can cause an imbalance that affects other glands, and when the hormonal system loses its equilibrium, it creates a negative protein balance of the body. But the glands also have a compensating factor that operates among them. There are instances where at least part of the function of a failing gland can be taken over by one or more of the remaining healthy glands.

The pituitary and the adrenals are good examples of this. Both of them produce hormones that have actions similar to those secreted by the sex glands. When the ovaries or the testicles fail to function, or if they have been removed, the hormones from the pituitary and adrenals pinch-hit for them by taking over some of their functions. This kind of "teamwork" is of great value and emphasizes the importance of keeping *all* your glands in good condition.

How to Keep Your Glands Healthy

"Good, nourishing food benefits the glands as inevitably as it does the entire body," says Dr. Rubin. He advises a well-balanced diet composed of a variety of foods, "particularly the protective ones that nutritionists stress." Dr. Rubin speaks of the "direct linkage of protein with glandular efficiency" and reminds us that the sex glands, particularly the male, aid in building up protein reserves. *All your glands need an adequate supply of protein to maintain their efficiency, to insure that the sex glands actively build up protein reserves, and to avoid a negative protein balance of the body.*

Here are other specific needs of certain glands:

Special Needs of the Pituitary

A healthy pituitary gives you an excellent chance of retaining youthful appearance, steady nerves, strong bones and keen mental powers well into old age. The vitamins most important for the health of this master gland are the B complex and vitamin E.

A deficiency of B complex causes a deterioration of the pituitary that affects other glandular functions, including those of the sex glands. Men are particularly vulnerable to such a deficiency. A lack of B vitamins results in a form of degeneration of the testes, though the ovaries escape damage. The posterior pituitary aids in regulating the water balance of the body, so it requires an adequate amount of water. The mineral most essential to its health is manganese, found abundantly in dark-green leafy vegetables.

Special Needs of the Adrenals

These glands of survival, discussed in an earlier chapter, are especially susceptible to nutritional deficiencies. They are easily damaged by undernourishment, by any diseases that throw poisons into the bloodstream, and by lead, nicotine and other chemicals.

To keep the adrenals in good health, be sure to include plenty of protein in the diet, along with foods rich in vitamin A, B complex, and perhaps most important of all, vitamin C. The adrenal cortex is a storehouse for large amounts of vitamin C, which is believed to aid in some way the gland's production of cortisone. Magnesium is the mineral most beneficial to the adrenals, and here again the dark-green leafy vegetables are the best source.

Special Needs of the Thyroid

Several years ago Dr. Louis Berman, a famous endocrinologist, succinctly described the vital functions of the thyroid, and what another authority called "its close and sympathetic relationship" with the sex glands of both men and women. Here is what he said:

> Without the thyroid there can be no complexity of thought, no learning, no education, no habit formation, no responsive energy for situations as well as no physical unfolding of faculty and function. *No reproduction of kind, with no sign of adolescence at the expected age and no exhibition of sex tendencies thereafter.* (My italics)

The thyroid has been called our pace maker. Thyroxin, the hormone it produces, regulates metabolism and governs the tempo at which body activities occur. When the thyroid fails to produce enough thyroxin, a person loses interest in sex. And even if he didn't, he wouldn't have the energy for it! An underactive thyroid (hypothyroidism) slows him down, mentally, physically, sexually. Both extremes—whether sluggish or overactive—cause the thyroid to produce too much thyroxin. Neither extreme is desirable.

Most of you probably know that iodine is essential to thyroid health. But a deficiency of vitamin E decreases the thyroid's absorption of iodine to five percent of normal. And when vitamin C is lacking, thyroxin is inactivated by oxygen. Protein is needed to supply the amino acid, tyrosine, from which thyroxin is made. And one of the B vitamins, choline, is essential for the production of thyroxin. Then, before the hormone can be used effectively, vitamins B_6 and C are necessary. These are just a few of the reasons why *all* the essential nutrients are advised for glandular health!

The pituitary, the adrenals and the thyroid are the glands known to be associated in various ways with sexual vigor and/or the sex glands themselves. There is not enough time to go into the functions of other glands that are less relevant to the present subject. But here, in summary, are their special nutritional needs.

The parathyroids must have calcium and vitamin D to keep them in good condition.

The thymus' main requirement is the B vitamin group. Its primary mineral need is chlorine.

The pancreas, like all the glands, needs a protein-rich diet, low in fats and starches which overburden it. Production of its most important hormone, insulin, is stimulated by B vitamins and the mineral zinc.

We now come to the glands most important to this discussion, the sex glands themselves.

Special Needs of the Gonads

Experiments have shown that young, virile men soon lost all interest in sex when they were kept on diets very low in protein. And in controlled tests, animals deprived of protein refused to mate. The vitamins most essential for healthy sex glands are A, B, C, E and F (the fatty acids). Iron and copper are the minerals most vital to their functioning.

Vitamin A assists the testes and ovaries by keeping the mucous membranes in good condition. Vitamins A and E are also beneficial in preventing prostate trouble, while three amino acids, glycine, alanine and glutamic acid, have been effective in curing enlarged prostate. (See page 136 for food sources of these three amino acids.)

A Japanese researcher, Dr. M. Higuchi, recently found that there is a relationship between vitamin C levels and hormone production of the sex glands! According to his research, the older person whose hormone production has slowed down needs much larger amounts of vitamin C than the younger person. Although vitamin C benefits the ovaries, men seem to have a greater need for it than women to keep their sex glands functioning well as they age.

The production of sex hormones stops if protein, several of the B vitamins, vitamin E and the fatty acids are lacking, and a serious deficiency of B_6 has been known to cause impotency. Vitamin D, which is chemically related to the sex hormones, is reported to have a stimulating effect on sexual drive.

Lecithin is an essential constituent of both the male and female sex glands. I have already recommended it for women, but because of his special problems, a man's need for it is even greater. Some thirty years ago, German doctors began using lecithin to treat male sexual debility, glandular exhaustion and other disorders. For almost as many years, I have personally recommended this vital food supplement to improve virility, aid the prevention of impotency, and for numerous other reasons that will be mentioned later.

Foods That Increase Sexual Vigor

There are foods that will have the effect of increasing sexual desire and ability. Anyone who has witnessed the therapeutic value of protein, vitamins, minerals, lecithin, desiccated liver and other concentrated food supplements in cases of sexual debility could not doubt it.

But if you're looking for a single food that packs the wallop of a powerful, instant aphrodisiac, the answer is no. Psychologists, doctors, nutritionists and sexologists agree that sustained sexual vigor depends upon the health of your body, glands and emotions. Their consistent health does not depend upon a single food, no matter how potent it is, but upon a combination of foods high in protein, vitamins and minerals. Added to that should be whatever concentrated food supplements are needed to counteract specific conditions and deficiencies.

TEN BASIC FOODS RECOMMENDED TO MAINTAIN HEALTH AND SEXUAL VIGOR

1. Meat
2. Fish
3. Poultry
4. Eggs
5. Whole grains (bread or cereal)
6. Milk products
7. Fresh fruit

8. Leafy green vegetables
9. Yellow vegetables
10. Unsaturated vegetable oils

These are all familiar, everyday foods. Giving them priority in your diet will help protect your health and vigor.

The foods on the next list are not staples in the average diet, but eating them often gives special benefits.

TEN SPECIAL FOODS THAT BENEFIT SEXUAL RESPONSE AND VIGOR

1. Liver (fresh or desiccated)
2. Lecithin
3. Oysters
4. Snails
5. Avocado
6. Sesame seeds
7. Honey (especially combined with sesame seeds)
8. Sprouted seeds and grains
9. Brewer's yeast
10. Wheat germ oil

Some of these foods and supplements are well known to my readers. But let's take a quick look at a few of them and see just what properties they possess that benefit sexual vigor.

Liver is one of the richest sources of vitamin B_{12}. Both the uterus and the seminal fluid contain a concentration of B_{12}, which seems to be important to their functioning. A lack of sexual interest and vigor has been noted in vegetarians who are deficient in B_{12}.

Folklore has long given credit to oysters for the prevention of impotency. Now scientists have found that the legend is based at least partly on fact. Oysters are an extremely rich source of the mineral zinc, and of the three amino acids mentioned earlier: glycine, alanine and glutamic acid. A shortage of zinc and the three amino acids is closely involved in the deterioration of the prostate gland. By correcting the deficiencies, doctors have been successful in restoring health to the prostate.

OTHER FOOD SOURCES OF ZINC

If you don't like oysters, you can still get enough zinc in liver, milk, wheat bran and wheat germ. But if you never eat liver, won't drink milk and always eat white bread, you're inviting a zinc deficiency—and possible prostate trouble.

BEST FOOD SOURCES OF GLYCINE, ALANINE, GLUTAMIC ACID

As you might expect, high-protein foods contain the greatest amount of these and other amino acids. The eight best sources of the three necessary for prostate health are:

1. Beef, lean
2. Liver, all kinds
3. Brewer's yeast
4. Casein (milk protein)
5. Milk, powdered skim
6. Veal, lean
7. Soybeans
8. Peanuts

Several centuries ago, women in Babylon ate candies made of sesame seeds and honey to improve their sexual responsiveness and fertility. The same type of candy is still available today in many stores, especially health food stores, but the legend has been almost forgotten. Let's see if it has any basis in fact.

Recently French research scientists found that the potassium and magnesium salts of aspartic acid were greatly beneficial in restoring vitality to women. An American doctor, P. E. Formica, has treated hundreds of women with the same formula and had a positive response in eighty-seven percent of his patients. An analysis of sesame seed candy shows that honey is rich in aspartic acid and sesame seeds in magnesium and potassium. Simmered together, they produce an excellent source of the potassium and magnesium salts of aspartic acid!

Snails are the only food known that contains pure glycogen (a form of sugar that has undergone several chemical processes in the liver before being stored to be released as the body needs it). In addition to supplying other vital needs, glycogen is an important element in the manufacture of male seminal fluid.

Both avocados and wheat germ oil are good sources of vitamin E. Wheat germ oil also contains appreciable amounts of estrogen in a natural form which boosts a woman's basic femininity if her own production of the hormone has slowed down. (Another food source of estrogen is hops. Though used mainly for brewing beer, it can also be used to brew a cup of vitalizing tea!)

Vitamin E has been called the fertility vitamin and the vitamin that puts new life into old love. Doctors who have prescribed it often admit to amazing results. Drs. Evan and Wilbur Shute of London, Ontario, Canada, hold an unchallenged record in vitamin E research. The Shute Vitamin E Institute has treated more than 30,000 patients with vitamin E. (Chapter 15 tells of their years of success in treating heart disease.) Dr. Evan Shute, fellow of the Royal Society of Surgeons and head of the institute that bears his name, says this about vitamin E and sexual vigor:

> Men have come here ostensibly suffering from impotence—they've come here after undergoing dangerous operations on their sex organs, after having taken all sorts of aphrodisiac drugs—then we've given them a simple vitamin—(the alpha tocopherol form of vitamin E)—and they're restored to normal sexual health.

Dr. Shute admits that doctors don't know why vitamin E cures impotence, then goes on to say, ". . . but we are sure that it is only a vitamin and hence can do no harm . . . We only know that it works." There is even the possibility that vitamin E may benefit the man whose impotence is psychologically induced. If it can give him confidence that his vigor will be restored, his original fear of failure that blocked adequate sexual performance may be removed.

You don't need false stimulants or exotic foods to improve your sexual desire and vigor. What you do need is the health that natural, protective foods can give you, with vitamins, minerals and other food supplements added as needed. Those who enjoy steak—and who doesn't?—may like to hear that Havelock Ellis, the famous sexologist, considered beefsteak "probably as powerful a sexual stimulant as any food." There can be no doubt that foods high in protein and rich in all the recommended vitamins and minerals form the basis of a virility diet for men and women of all ages. As British author Barbara Cartland said, "If every woman fed her husband two pounds of good red meat every day, there wouldn't be any need for all these 'dirty films'!"

A protein-rich diet will also do much toward keeping the heart alive, insuring that arterial walls remain as free as possible from fatty deposits and that the heart is not burdened by high blood fat and cholesterol levels. Those people who continue to eat foods with high fat and sugar content must beware of heart trouble.

14

Danger! Heart at Work

There is a dangerous killer in America that strikes down an average of 1,900 persons a day. Its name is *atherosclerosis.* Cholesterol is its chief accomplice. It takes its toll in heart attacks and cerebral brain strokes. Heart attacks account for 1,400 of the 1,900 daily deaths—with more than a death a minute every twenty-four hours! And, within the same time period, cerebral brain strokes take another 500 lives.

Atherosclerosis is a form of *arteriosclerosis,* or hardening of the arteries. Sometimes you hear the two words used interchangeably, but there is a difference between them that can mean the difference between life and death. Arteriosclerosis may or may not be accompanied by a blockage within the artery that can trigger a stroke or a heart attack. Atherosclerosis invariably produces some measure of narrowing and blockage within the artery.

Arteriosclerosis is the hardening of the arteries that takes place in varying degrees in everyone, from birth until death (even in the embryo, to a certain extent). Many persons in their seventies and eighties show only a slight evidence of it while, in the same age group, some will have extensive hardening in one set of arteries and very little in the others. The most vital arteries are the ones that seem to be particularly subject to hardening as we grow older. They are the aorta (the large artery that carries blood from the heart to be distributed by branch arteries through the body) and the arteries supplying the heart, brain, liver, kidneys and legs.

In *atherosclerosis,* deposits of cholesterol and other fatty substances accumulate on the artery wall. When they accumulate in amounts so large that the artery walls are unable to dispose of them, the fat-loaded cells break down. In a series of biological processes that include the overburdened cells' release of the fatty substances, the irritation of neighboring cells and the formation of scar tissue, the artery wall hardens, thickens, and its passageway narrows. This is a type of biological "rust" comparable to the rust that forms inside a water pipe and eventually slows down or chokes off the flow from the faucet. Biological rust can slow down, block or choke off the flow of blood to the heart, brain and other parts of the body, depending on which arteries are narrowed or blocked.

A partial blockage that restricts the blood supply to the brain may result in confusion, loss of mental acuity and memory, premature senility—or a stroke.

The walls of normal arteries are smooth, supple and flexible. Their elastic quality enables them to contract and expand so that the blood can flow freely through them. In the four major types of heart disease, the coronary arteries (those supplying blood to the heart) are to a greater or lesser extent narrowed and blocked with fatty substances.

The fatty substances that cause blockage in sclerotic arteries consist largely of cholesterol. A high blood cholesterol is not the only cause of strokes and heart attacks. *But by remembering that the basic atherosclerosis is involved in all of them, you can do a great deal to protect yourself.* (You'll find out how as we go along.)

Such a variety of heart disorders results from atherosclerosis that the term "hardening of the arteries" is sometimes loosely used to describe the full range. All of them result from a restricted blood flow through the coronary arteries. Each one merely shows different stages and manifestations of the same underlying conditions.

Four Major Heart Diseases

1. *Coronary occlusion, or thrombosis:* This attack can strike suddenly, sometimes with little or no warning. A coronary occlusion occurs when severe atherosclerosis causes a blockage within a coronary artery that shuts off the supply of oxygen and nourishment to a certain area of the heart. Since fatty substances accumulate slowly on the artery walls, it may take years for this type of blockage to build up. As children, we have the ability to absorb the fatty deposits that fasten themselves to our artery walls. But at some undetermined time between youth and maturity this power of absorption is lost, and with it, the body's natural protection against coronary-artery disease. By the time an American male is twenty-five, his arteries usually show sizable deposits of cholesterol and other fats.

A former president of the American Heart Association, Howard Sprague, maintains that at least forty percent of all American men over forty years of age have a substantial degree of obstruction in their arteries. And that for men between forty and sixty-two, the death rate is alarmingly high.

There is a greater tendency for clots to form in the blood of persons who have atherosclerosis, even in those whose cases are not advanced. Blockage from a *thrombus,* or blood clot, takes only minutes to form, and the result may be rapidly fatal. When a thrombus or other blockage shuts off the blood flow to the heart, there is death of some tissue and cells in a segment of heart muscle. This condition is known as *myocardial infarction,* and before the patient can recover, time must be given for the destroyed area to be filled in with normal tissue. Recovery usually means from two to six weeks of rest in bed, depending upon the severity of the attack. Coronary thrombosis has become a major killer of progressively younger men each year.

2. *Angina pectoris:* The recurring pains of angina pectoris are usually centered beneath the breastbone or over the heart region on the left side. The pain often travels down the left arm, sometimes as far as the ring and little fingers. It occurs when narrowed or constricted arteries are unable to allow the passage

of sufficient blood and oxygen to reach a certain segment of heart muscle. When this happens, the heart muscle develops a painful spasm, or "cramp," which comes on suddenly and lasts for several minutes.

Angina pectoris afflicts both young and old, and, as in other heart attacks, atherosclerosis, overweight and prolonged high blood pressure are major predisposing factors. Since most persons suffering from angina have some degenerative changes within the artery, the condition may be a forerunner of coronary thrombosis. An attack of angina may be provoked by excessive cigarette smoking, eating too much and too fast, overexertion, emotional upsets, excitement or severe stress.

3. *Acute coronary insufficiency,* like angina, involves failure of the coronary artery. In angina, the blood supply to the heart may be adequate when at rest but insufficient when under certain conditions the heart is required to pump harder and its nutritive requirements increase. Acute coronary insufficiency is more severe and the pain more persistent, because blood flow to the active heart muscle is impaired. Damage to the heart muscle is generally restricted to a particular localized segment. The insufficiency is almost always brought on by blockage of a small artery due to atherosclerosis, plus a spasm of the artery.

Heart failure, or cardiac decomposition: Heart failure has a frightening and final sound. But it doesn't mean that the heart has failed completely. Although its efficiency as a pump is impaired and it can no longer perform the normal work it once did, it doesn't just suddenly stop. When it becomes weakened by its own failure to receive an adequate supply of blood, the heart muscle in turn fails to pump sufficient blood to all the body tissues. Some of the symptoms of heart failure are these:

The need to sleep propped up with pillows in a semisitting position,

A chronic cough,

Shortness of breath during mild exertion or even while resting or talking,

An irregular pulse and heartbeat and

Swelling of the legs and ankles, especially toward the end of the day.

If chronic heart failure has severely damaged the heart muscle, it may be necessary to keep the patient in bed for a few weeks. To prevent an abnormal retention of fluid in the tissues, consumption of salt and liquids is restricted.

In heart failure, atherosclerosis is again the prime suspect. Other contributing causes include severe anemia, rheumatic heart disease that damages the heart valves, extensive liver, kidney and lung disease (emphysema, tuberculosis, and bronchiectasis) and bacterial infection in the heart valves.

Although the initial damage to the heart cannot be repaired, victims of heart failure may live comparatively long and comfortable lives by taking these precautions:

1. Stay thin. If overweight, reduce.

2. Keep the diet *high* in protein, vitamins and minerals, and *low* in fats and starches—*especially animal fats.*

3. Limit the use of spices. Restrict the salt intake and the amount of liquids consumed to prevent edema (sometimes called dropsy), the excessive accumulation of fluid in the tissues mentioned above.

4. Avoid catching cold. (Remember that plenty of protein and all the essential nutrients, with special emphasis on vitamins A and C, aid in building up your resistance to colds.) The studies of a British medical researcher, Dr. F. J. Flint, and recent reports in the *American Journal of Medical Science* and *Diuretic Review* give new evidence that respiratory infections, particularly colds, are among the most common aggravating factors in congestive heart failure. According to Dr. Flint, who studied hundreds of cases of heart failure, "respiratory infections in the person with a weak heart may initiate cardiac failure by causing damage to the heart muscle or by favoring congestion of the lungs."

Atherosclerosis is a forerunner of these and other heart conditions that involve some degree of blockage in the coronary arteries. Of them all, coronary thrombosis is the most dreaded. It has become the major cause of heart attacks—and sudden death—among four out of five men between the ages of forty to sixty. When a major artery suddenly closes, death often follows within minutes. I witnessed a tragic example of this in London.

An old friend of mine, Harry Jordan, met me for luncheon. I noticed that he had gained about thirty pounds since I last saw him, but he told me that he felt fine and had a hearty appetite. Much too hearty for his heart's sake, I soon found out. He started out with a double Scotch and soda, followed by a bowl of vichysoisse and several rolls slathered with butter. Next he had a large steak, which he ate fat and all, an order of fried potatoes and peas in cream sauce. For dessert he had chocolate pie with whipped cream.

He saw the look of concern on my face and said, "I know you think I'm eating too much. But I only had coffee for breakfast."

"I was trying to restrain myself," I told him. "But since you brought it up, you are eating too much—and all the wrong things! Besides, when you skip a meal, so much stored fat pours into the blood that it rises several times above normal. This can endanger the life of anyone subject to heart attacks."

"I know a chap who's a heart patient," he said. "Has to eat five or six small meals a day instead of large ones. Is that the reason?"

"It's one of the reasons. When you overeat, your cholesterol level rises. If you eat just the amount of food you need, it's influenced by how much fat your meals contain and whether the fats are saturated or unsaturated. When you eat a lot of the saturated fats—such as the fat on your steak and all the butter and cream you've just stowed away—the cholesterol level rises. But when you cut down on animal fats and increase the unsaturated fats (safflower, soybean, peanut and other vegetable oils) in your diet, the cholesterol level falls. By the way, have you ever had a test to find out how high your blood cholesterol is?"

"No reason to," he said. "Nothing wrong with me except an occasional twinge of indigestion."

"You know I'm not an alarmist, Harry," I said. "But unless you cut down on your total calories, especially fat and sugar, get a little exercise and take off some weight, I'm afraid you're in danger of having a heart attack or a stroke."

"Who, me?" A laugh as hearty as the meal he had eaten shook his large abdomen. "Why, I've never been sick a day in my life."

The next time we met, as we were walking from the restaurant, Harry suddenly clutched frantically at his chest, and his eyes filled with pain and terror. He slumped forward, and I lowered him to the sidewalk. An ambulance came, but it was too late. It was Harry's first and last heart attack. His death was a shocking and tragic loss to his family and friends. But the saddest part of it was that it could have been prevented. Harry's high-fat-and-sugar diet, his overweight and physically inactive life had been mainly responsible for making him a heart attack victim at an early age.

Your way of living and eating can make *you* heart-attack-prone—unless you recognize the predisposing factors and learn how to protect your heart.

You Are Heart-Attack-Prone *If* . . .

If even two or three of the following risk factors are present, your chances of having a heart attack before you're sixty-five become one in two:

1. Marked atherosclerosis.
2. High cholesterol levels, especially over a period of time.
3. Overweight. If you're fat, you run a fifty percent greater risk of having a heart attack or a stroke than those of normal weight.
4. Overeating, *especially* of foods high in animal fats and sugar. But don't let your *total* calorie intake go too high either. Fatness is a measure of overeating—and the death rate rises and falls with the degree of overweight.
5. Chronically high blood pressure.
6. Diabetes.
7. Excessive cigarette smoking.
8. Physical inactivity.

You should be able to control six of these risk factors yourself with the right diet, will power and moderate exercise.

You Can Protect Your Heart *If* . . .

If you *reverse* the risk factors, your chances of having a heart attack before sixty-five are only one in twenty to one in fifty. *You should be able to qualify for the heart-saving odds if you:*

1. Make a practice of eating the foods that help prevent atherosclerosis. Add to your daily diet the supplements—lecithin, in particular—that have in many cases reversed atherosclerosis.
2. Keep your blood cholesterol at an average or low level. The best levels are under 200, or if possible, under 175, but not many middle-aged American men ever achieve the latter. A reading above 250 is definitely high, though the average for men between forty-five and sixty-five in this country runs between 230 and 240.
3. Keep your weight and blood pressure normal.
4. Don't smoke. If you can't stop, cut down as much as possible. The coronary risk is three to six times greater in cigarette smokers than it is in nonsmokers.
5. Avoid diabetes by keeping the pancreas functioning normally. (See page 67 for foods that keep it healthy.) Most important, don't overload it with sugar and other high carbohydrates. The danger of developing coronary disease is two to four times greater among diabetics than it is in those without it.
6. Stay physically active. The sedentary person runs twice the risk of coronary-artery disease than those who are physically active. Exercise seems to be of almost equal value in preventing a heart attack or in reconditioning the person who has had one.

Exercises to Protect Your Heart

Leading heart specialists from all parts of the world are in agreement with Dr. Edward Bortz, who said, "If American men would accept an exercise program as a regular part of their lives, in three to five years we could cut the coronary death rate in half." Persons who exercise not only have far fewer heart attacks than those who are inactive, but when one does occur, it is usually less severe and the chances of recovery are much better.

"Five minutes of exercise a day may prevent death from atherosclerosis!" This was the report made by a Cologne University cardiology and sports medicine professor, Dr. Wildor Hollman, at the 16th Annual Congress for Sports Medicine in Hanover, Germany.

Prevention is also emphasized in Russia, where factory workers stop work every forty-five minutes and take an exercise break, according to Dr. Fedor Romashov, a U.S.S.R. Medical Chief. It should be noted that Russia is not included among the nations that lead the world death rates for heart disease. The United States is first on that lethal list, with Finland, Canada, Australia, New Zealand, England and West Germany the runners-up.

But for those who already have advanced atherosclerosis, Dr. William B. Kannel of Harvard University gives these words of hope: "Persons who have an important degree of blockage of the coronary artery, but continue physically active, can reasonably be expected to develop more collateral circulation [branch arteries] than those with comparable coronary involvement who remain inactive."

A condensed report on coronary blockage made by Dr. Edgar Rentoul of Houston, Renfrewshire, England, to *The Lancet* corroborates the importance of exercise for a healthy heart:

> (a) The bigger the coronary arteries, the more room there is to have atheromatous plaques without disastrous results. (b) The part played by exercise is clear. The more you exercise, the bigger your coronary arteries, the faster the blood goes through them, [and] the more difficult it is for an obstruction to develop on the walls.

The experts all agree that exercises to protect the heart must be vigorous enough to give the heart and lungs a good workout and create an expanded capillary network. The new capillaries created by this type of exercise supplement the blood supply to the heart endangered by atherosclerosis. They also agree that low-tension sports are best for the middle-aged sedentary man (or woman), and that even these should be started at an easy, moderate pace, gradually working up to more vigorous activity. Most people are not prepared for the high-tension sports that require bursts of intensive activity—at least not until they've conditioned themselves.

At the other extreme are the sports *too* low-tension to expand the capillaries and prevent the blockage of arteries. Golf, bowling and volley ball aren't vigorous enough to improve your heart and blood vessel function and to lower your blood cholesterol. The exercises described below have been chosen to do exactly that.

Walking. Dr. Paul Dudley White recommends walking for everyone. "The easiest exercise of all," he says, "requiring no equipment except shoe leather." Now in his eighties and still a champion walker, he suggests a five-mile walk a day, with arms relaxed and swinging and some good, deep breaths taken along the way.

Harvard's Dr. Frederick Stare is another famous walking enthusiast, but his prescription for beginners is less strenuous. "Walk for ten to fifteen minutes once a day," he says, "at a moderately brisk pace. Promote yourself gradually until you reach a brisk twenty-minute walk three times a day."

Is walking the only exercise necessary to protect your heart? A member of the Council on Arteriosclerosis of the American Heart Association believes that it is, *if you start early enough and keep it up vigorously and consistently*.

"Vigorous walking," says Dr. M. F. Graham of the University of Texas Southwestern Medical School, "if practiced from youth on, would in itself reduce the disability and early deaths due to coronary heart disease."

Jogging. Walking and jogging (or running) are given priority because, as Dr. White says, they don't require any special equipment, skill or technique. If you're unable to jog outdoors, you can jog in place, as described in Chapter 12. Jogging has become the single most popular conditioner. Heart specialists prescribe it to prevent heart attacks and as a reconditioner for people who have had heart attacks. It is an easy, pleasant way to condition the entire body and to promote mental alertness.

Watch the early-morning joggers in Washington, D.C., and you'll recognize many familiar faces. The handsome couple jogging together—and wearing his and her black nylon sweat suits—are Senator and Mrs. Mark Hatfield of Oregon. Other famous joggers include Attorney General and Mrs. Ramsey Clark and Senator William Proxmire of Wisconsin, who jogs a total of nine miles a day to and from the Capitol.

Brisk walking and jogging, or easy running, help lower blood cholesterol, prevent atherosclerosis, build up branch arteries to supplement those that are blocked, and develop greater endurance in the heart, lungs, and muscles. So will bicycling, swimming, and rowing. Rowing is last on the list because, although it benefits the heart and lungs, it doesn't increase the endurance of the entire body, as do the others.

Like the air you breathe, exercise cannot be purchased in containers to be used when the mood strikes you. Breathing, of course, is an automatic function, while exercise is often a chore—until you train your body to accept it on a regular basis.

Exercise may be said to be the mechanical care of the heart (and body). Of equal importance is the food with which the heart is nourished. The next chapter is devoted to a study of the food elements that optimally condition the heart and the best sources of these elements.

15

Eating to Keep Your Heart Alive

"You are what you eat" is an often-heard cliché, particularly true where the heart is concerned. Good nutrition is important to prevent or forestall heart disease. Since we know that certain foods have a negative, potentially disastrous effect on the heart, now is the time to analyze your eating habits. You may spot a few warning signs. The time to modify bad eating habits is while you are healthy enough to do so, *before* degeneration sets in. Knowing what to do—and doing it—can add many years of effective usefulness to your heart's life. Because cholesterol is one of the heart's enemies, let's begin with that.

What You Eat Can Raise or Lower Your Cholesterol Level

In compiling their portrait of an average American male headed for a heart attack, the Framingham Heart Study of Framingham, Massachusetts, investigated more than 5,000 cases. Their composite portrait was of a middle-aged sedentary "given to excessive cigarette smoking and to *meals high in animal fats, sugar and cholesterol.*" (My italics)

This doesn't mean that you should cut out all foods that contain animal fats and cholesterol. You couldn't do it, anyway, unless you existed on a substandard diet—and then you wouldn't exist very long. *But you can and should reduce your intake of them as much as possible.*

When you eat large amounts of foods high in animal fats and cholesterol, these fats work together to raise the blood cholesterol levels. By making the following substitutions in your diet, you can lower your cholesterol and other blood fats to a normal level.

Avoid These Foods:

High-fat meats (and trim away all visible fat on the lean cuts), luncheon meats, pizza and high-fat cheese.

All fried foods, lard and other hard cooking fats.

Gravies, cream sauces and rich salad dressing.

Butter and margarine (except in *very* limited amounts, and then only if combined half and half with safflower or other unsaturated oil).

Hot breads (and the butter you'd pile on them).

Casseroles and stews cooked in cream sauce and gravy.

Creamed soups, creamed vegetables and other creamed foods.

Whipped cream, whole milk and the usual commercial ice cream.

Chocolate in *any* form.

Pie, cake, cookies, sweet rolls and all bakery goods high in both sugar and fats. (You can make them yourself with wholesome ingredients.)

Substitute These Foods:

Lean meats and poultry, ocean fish and seafood. (Try to have fish several times a week.)

Bake, broil, grill or roast the above foods (fish may also be steamed or poached in white wine, skim milk or tomato juice) or sauté them in a little safflower or other vegetable oil.

Use vegetable oils instead of hard (saturated) fats for all cooking. The *best* is safflower oil.

All vegetables cooked without cream or butter or eaten raw in salads.

Use salad dressing made of safflower oil and lemon juice or vinegar.

Consommé, bouillon, vegetable, tomato or other low-fat soups made without cream, butter or meat fat.

Skim milk, low-fat milk, buttermilk or reconstituted powdered skim milk.

Ices and sherbets made without cream and sweetened with honey instead of sugar.

Yogurt, low-fat cheese.

All fresh fruit, melons and berries. Dried fruit occasionally.

What about eggs? You've probably heard that they contain cholesterol, and they do. For that reason, some doctors omit them from their patients' diets. But many nutritionists and heart specialists do not agree. One of the world's greatest heart surgeons, Dr. Michael Ellis de Bakey of Methodist Hospital, Houston, Texas, calls the omission of eggs from the diet "a fad diet." "An egg a day is OK," he says and only cautions, "Don't eat them three times a day."

A nine-year study reported by Dr. Edward H. Ahrens of the Rockefeller Institute revealed that for persons who ate, at a single meal, twelve eggs fried in peanut oil, their cholesterol levels didn't increase. But when they ate twelve eggs fried in saturated fats, the rise in cholesterol was high and rapid. In the same experiments it was discovered that patients kept on a diet containing *no fat at all* had the highest blood-fat levels, while those who ate normal amounts of *predominantly unsaturated fats* had the lowest. A certain amount of fat is essential for health, and when you omit all fats from your diet, stored fat pours into the bloodstream, as it does when you skip a meal.

The important facts to remember are these:

1. *Safflower, soybean, peanut, corn and other unsaturated oils tend to lower the blood-fat and cholesterol levels.*

2. *The saturated, or animal, fats cause the blood-fat and cholesterol levels to rise.*

A good general rule to follow is one recommended by researchers from Canada (the Canadian Heart Foundation), the United States, England and India, who together tested more than 1,000 men: *One-half to two-thirds of the total fat in your diet should be unsaturated.*

A vital reason for this is that in the absence of three fatty acids —linoleic, linolenic and arachadonic—animal (saturated) fats are unable to burn as they should and accumulate in the blood. Unsaturated vegetable oils are the best source of fatty acids. By making sure that they outweigh the animal fats in your diet, the damage caused by an excess of animals fats can be prevented.

Sugar and Your Heart

When you eat an excess of high carbohydrate foods, what is not burned as calories is rapidly changed into saturated fats, causing a rapid rise in cholesterol and blood fat. More calories than your body can burn and too much of any refined carbohydrate, including alcohol, will have this effect. My advice for many years has been, "Cut down on high-starch foods; cut out sugar—and don't overeat anything!"

But sugar is the worst offender. Today's statistics show that fifty percent of the average American diet consists of refined sugar and flour products. And *that* is considered normal!

When you figure the large number of diabetics, hypoglycemics, and others who are allowed no sugar at all, it doesn't take a mathematician to see that a big percentage of Americans are eating dangerous amounts of sugar, dangerous because refined sugar is a nutritional death trap. It commits a great sin against health by drawing from the body significant amounts of residue body-mineral content, thus robbing it of vital elements it had before the sugar was consumed.

Dr. John Yudkin of the University of London is noted for his outstanding research linking sugar with heart disease. His tests, reported in *The Lancet* and other scientific and medical journals, have shown that patients with advanced atherosclerosis and coronary-artery disease ate twice as much sugar as those whose arteries were normal. Also writing in *The Lancet,* Dr. T.

L. Cleave, former surgeon captain of the Royal Navy of Great Britain, blames *two* refined carbohydrates for causing artery and heart disease: white sugar and white flour.

Drs. Cheraskin, Ringsdorf and Clark of the University of Alabama have reported evidence that eating *any* amount of "simple carbohydrates such as refined sugar increases the blood cholesterol level significantly." They point out that eating *complex* carbohydrates (those called natural) as found in fresh fruits, vegetables, whole grains, potatoes and legumes, can actually *reduce* the blood cholesterol.

Another team of experts headed by Drs. Willard A. Krehl and Robert E. Hodges of the University of Iowa reported on the incidence of heart disease and its relation to dietary habits. They confirmed what many specialists, including Drs. Yudkin and Cleave, have said: It's the *type* of carbohydrates you eat that can make you a candidate for a heart attack—and that type is the *refined* carbohydrates—mainly white sugar and its byproducts!

British and American research have shown that sugar increases the danger of a coronary attack by building up fatty tissue on the walls of coronary arteries and by altering fat metabolism. It is no wonder that many big sugar eaters suffer from chronic fatigue and heart disturbances.

There is, of course, no sweetening material better than honey. It should always be used in preference to refined sugar. Honey is "oats for the heart"—its power supply.

Professor Dr. E. Koch, famous German heart specialist, most emphatically approves of honey for the heart: "The heart, after getting honey, can be compared with a horse after feeding it oats. It is loaded with strength."

Dr. G. N. W. Thomas of Edinburgh said in *The Lancet:* "In heart weaknesses, I have found honey to have a marked effect in reviving the heart action and keeping patients alive. I suggest honey should be given for general physical repair and, above all, for heart failure."

You may wonder how a simple, good-tasting sweet can serve as a wonderful food on the one hand and as nourishment for weakened heart muscles on the other. The explanation is that honey contains as its prime ingredient the sugar dextrose which is readily converted to glycogen by the body. Glycogen is the only form in which sugar can be stored in the human body (main storage places are the liver, gland cells, and muscles) for ready use whenever energy is needed or when exertion makes the heart pump extra hard.

In addition to honey, there are other food elements which are extremely beneficial, even essential, to the continued health of the heart and arteries.

Food Elements That Protect Your Heart

It seems that all the nutrients that benefit the body help in a direct or indirect way to prevent atherosclerosis—and thus decrease the danger of a heart attack. With certain nutrients, the process is slow and scarcely noticeable. But two of them are capable of giving a definite and often dramatic improvement within a matter of weeks. These two are the alpha tocopherol form of vitamin E and the food supplement lecithin.

Vitamin E

Vitamin E is an antithrombin. By retarding coagulation of the blood, it aids in the prevention of blood clots. When a blockage does occur, according to Drs. Wilbur and Evan Shute, vitamin E can produce new blood vessels around the obstruction, enabling the flow of blood to continue.

When given in large amounts, vitamin E has reduced blood cholesterol levels in many individuals. It improves the circulation, strengthens the heart muscle and capillaries, aids the body's use of oxygen and prevents oxygen starvation. The latter is a serious problem in coronary insufficiency. *Its oxygen-saving power and its ability to dilate the capillaries are major factors in preventing death from coronary thrombosis.*

The Drs. Shute have been treating heart patients with vitamin E for almost twenty-five years. They have had outstanding success with patients suffering from all types of heart disease, including the "despair" cases, victims of chronic rheumatic heart disease. The "despair" patients have congestive failure and other complications, are often bedfast, and can take practically no exercise. "Yet we have had patients in this category," the Shutes report, "who had spent six to nineteen months in bed under classical therapy, who were able to resume full activity and maintain normal living with increasing strength. This has occurred in as little as a month on alpha tocopherol (vitamin E) treatment . . ." They have found that "the key to success depends upon fitting the dosage to the individual's peculiar requirements." (*The Summary,* 12:67)

Their years of experience have shown them that many persons fail to get results because they don't take enough. (They consider amounts less than 50 to 100 units in the "no-result" category which discourages a patient and causes him to stop the treatment.) Their usual prescription is many times that amount, except for certain patients with high blood pressure or chronic rheumatic heart disease and evidence of congestive failure. For the first few weeks these patients are put on small amounts, with the dosage gradually increased. The dosage can range across a broad scale. At the Shute Institute, the chronic rheumatic heart disease patients are treated cautiously, beginning with 90 units a day and gradually increasing it until their optimum is reached.

For coronary attacks, the Shutes believe that maximum help should be given as quickly as possible. Although in many cases a smaller amount is adequate, to avoid unnecessary risk they feel that coronary patients should immediately be given 1,600 units.

In between the two extremes is the angina pectoris patient. If no other cardiac complications are present, he is given 800 units a day. In most cases, an improvement is evident within six weeks, and the patient is kept on that amount as a maintenance dose, because it was discovered that if the dosage is lowered following improvement, the symptoms soon recur.

There are some angina patients, the Shutes say, who will show no improvement, even when the dosage is increased 200 units every six weeks by their customary procedure for patients slow to respond. The patients slow to improve and those who show no response at all both are kept on a maintenance dose of 800 units a day to prevent the ever-present possibility of an attack of coronary thrombosis.

Many doctors who are just beginning to treat heart patients with vitamin E have told me that although their experimental use of it has been successful, they need guidelines to help determine the amounts to be administered. Only recently have the Shutes overcome their understandable reluctance to supply those guidelines.

And right here I want to remind you that the recommendations in this chapter are to *protect* your heart from danger. It should definitely be understood that the person who already has a heart condition is *not* being advised to treat himself. But what he *can* do, if he isn't being given vitamin E, is call its proven merits to his doctor's attention and ask for treatment with it according to the Drs. Shutes' recommended dosage.

The two doctors explain the tolerance for vitamin E this way: "A patient with a normal or low blood pressure and with no evidence of congestive failure can usually, but not quite always, tolerate any quantity of alpha tocopherol." They define the right dose as the one that produces a definite improvement in the patient, usually within four to six weeks. "The maintenance dose," says Dr. Evan Shute, "is the same."

For the person who has so far suffered little or no coronary artery damage but who wants to protect his heart from potential attacks, the usual recommendation for a daily maintenance dose is from 100 to 300 international units of the alpha tocopherol form of vitamin E.

Lecithin

"The furnace in which body fats are burned" is the definition given of lecithin as long ago as 1891. Lecithin is a powerful fat emulsifier, effective both as a preventive and as a remedy for atherosclerosis. It aids fat transportation, keeps it from settling down in dangerous places, and causes cholesterol and fats to be broken up into particles tiny enough to pass through the artery walls instead of accumulating on them.

In his book *The Low-Fat Way to Health and Longer Life,* Dr. Lester M. Morrison, senior attending physician, Los Angeles County General Hospital, describes lecithin as "one of our most powerful weapons against disease." Speaking of the many preparations he has used in his years of work in the treatment and prevention of heart and artery disease, he says: "We found lecithin to give the most rewarding result . . . It is an especially valuable bulwark against development of 'hardening of the arteries' [atherosclerosis] and all the complications of heart, brain and kidney that follow." He has found it effective not only in lowering cholesterol levels and *preventing* atherosclerosis and heart and artery disease, but in treating advanced cases of atherosclerosis and, in countless instances, even *reversing* atherosclerosis, making old, sclerotic arteries younger.

Dr. Morrison and other specialists cite evidence of lecithin's power to "melt away" plaques already deposited on arterial walls and to regenerate arteries partially blocked by advanced atherosclerosis.

Chemically classified as a *phospholipid,* lecithin is essential to every cell in the body. A high concentration of it is found in such vital organs as the heart, brain, kidneys, endocrine glands, and in the myelin sheath that surrounds and protects the nerve fibers. In healthy individuals, almost a third of the brain's weight is composed of lecithin, and more than twice that amount is found in the liver. In persons who have died of heart disease, autopsies have shown a great decrease in the lecithin content of vital organs.

Lecithin is a rich source of food elements that give exceptional protection to your heart and arteries. It contains the fatty acids, vitamin E, and choline and inositol, two B vitamins that are potent fat-dissolving agents. It also provides significant amounts of other nutrients essential for health, including vitamins A, D and K.

Lecithin increases the gamma globulin content of the blood, which aids in building up the protective forces of the body. In this way, lecithin increases immunity against all virus infections, from colds to pneumonia. Lecithin's proved benefits are applicable to a long list of conditions—possibly even including the prevention of such diseases as infectious hepatitis or at least reducing the severity of attacks that do occur.

Vitamins and Minerals for a Healthy Heart

Vitamin A: When heart patients were given 100,000 units of vitamin A daily for three to six months, the lecithin content of their bodies showed a definite increase, and their cholesterol level fell to normal.

B complex: A deficiency of *vitamin* B_1 and *pantothenic acid* can damage the heart muscles and impair the circulation. The resulting condition increases the danger of blood clotting. Add vitamin B_6 to *choline, inositol* and *lecithin,* and these substances function as effective agents in utilizing fats, lowering cholesterol and preventing or reversing atherosclerosis.

For lecithin to be synthesized in the body, *vitamin* B_6 and the mineral *magnesium* must be present. Five hundred milligrams of magnesium a day has been used successfully to reverse severe atherosclerosis and lower cholesterol levels within a matter of weeks. By stepping up the body's production of bile salts, *vitamin* B_{12} causes a reduction in the amounts of cholesterol in the bloodstream.

Vitamin C helps vitamin E provide oxygen for the heart and works to prevent or fight off infections. The *vitamin C complex* (a combination of *vitamin C, rutin,* and the nutrients extracted from citrus known as the *bioflavonoids*) strengthens fragile capillaries and has been used successfully to prevent the "little strokes" that ultimately lead to major ones. Evidence of vitamin C's usefulness in reducing cholesterol levels has been reported in *Nutrition News* (7:64) and other publications. In tests with animals, those deprived of vitamin C produced cholesterol six times faster than the nondeficient animals.

In other experiments, Dr. Hans Selye, the noted authority on stress, found that all the test animals subjected to severe stress developed serious heart disease—except those that had potassium and magnesium added to their diets! Both *magnesium* and *potassium* protect the heart and brain by helping to prevent the formation of clots. Without potassium in the diet, dead tissue soon develops within the heart muscles. (A suggested way to increase your potassium intake, reduce your salt intake—and lessen the risk of high blood pressure—is to fill your saltshaker with equal amounts of potassium-chloride salt and sea salt.)

Calcium: From Japan comes scientific research that calcium is effective in preventing disorders of the blood vessels and certain abnormalities of the heart and brain. Six scientists at the Tohoku University School of Medicine decided to investigate the high incidence of death from heart attacks and strokes in soft-water areas of Japan compared with the low incidence in regions where people drank and cooked with hard, mineral-rich water. Their series of experiments, published in the *Tohoku Journal of Experimental Medicine,* gave evidence that a calcium deficiency is a contributing cause to the prevalence of high blood pressure and death from strokes.

When calcium is deficient, the heart beats faster, is unable to relax, and the heart muscle is impaired. Calcium has been used in congestive heart failure since the beginning of this century. American scientists have also known for some years the value of hard, mineralized water in maintaining heart and artery health. Part of the reason mineralized water is so beneficial also has to do with the "trace" minerals it contains.

Trace minerals: A number of the trace minerals supplied by hard water and certain foods help provide protection from heart and artery disease. *Chromium, zinc* and *vanadium* are the most important of these trace minerals. Dr. William H. Strain, of the University of Rochester's School of Medicine, is one of many researchers who believes that the amount of trace minerals contained in hard, mineral-rich water is a major factor in determining how long we will live.

Chromium helps protect the heart and arteries by keeping blood pressure normal. Research linking a deficiency of *zinc* with atherosclerosis has come from three American universities:

Harvard, University of Rochester Medical Center and the University of Missouri, as well as from the Minsk Medical Institute of Russia.

The four foods that contain the largest amounts of *zinc* are liver, milk, wheat germ and wheat bran. The best food sources of *vanadium* are sardines and herring (unsmoked and unsalted), although other ocean fish contain varying amounts of it. Traces of *chromium* are found in almost all soil and plant life. Since even the little-known trace minerals are essential for health, unless your diet includes plenty of leafy greens and raw fruit, it's a good policy to add a vitamin-mineral supplement to your diet. It's especially important if you live where the water is soft and deficient in minerals.

New benefits in everyday foods are constantly being discovered. A few years ago, Dr. Ancel Keys, American Heart Association physiologist, discovered that fifteen grams of pectin a day helps lower blood cholesterol. That's approximately the amount of pectin you get by eating two apples—so *two* apples a day may keep the heart doctor away!

Sex and the Heart Patient

Sooner or later, nearly all men who have had a heart attack will ask: "What about sex?" One doctor was reported to have advised a worried patient who posed this question to him, "It's all right, but only with your wife—I don't want you to get excited!" Dr. de Bakey gives essentially the same advice in these words: "A normal sex life is fine. The best advice: Maintain a balanced sex life, not a hysterical one."

For those who have already suffered a heart attack or a stroke, studies have shown that the patient with a positive outlook recovers far more rapidly than the one with a hopeless outlook. Dr. Paul Dudley White believes that "one should as early as possible develop an optimistic philosophy. To those already afflicted with heart disease," he says, "especially of a coronary nature, we have found in a long, follow-up study that many patients improve with the years and can actually outgrow their troubles . . . *if they cooperate with nature*."

To make your heart last for the more than 3,000,000,000 beats of a normal lifetime, Dr. White emphasizes an old but true maxim: *"An ounce of prevention is worth a pound of cure."* (My italics) "This time around, however," he says, "it is based on the most advanced scientific research into the factors that contribute to and cause heart disease in whole populations."

You have learned what those factors are, how to protect your heart and arteries from them, and how you can reverse some of the damage that may already exist. To keep your heart from stopping prematurely, two of its chief requirements are exercise and the right food to keep it healthy and to replenish its energy. But neither food nor exercise can be stored. They must be renewed every day. For your heart's sake, see that they are.

16

What the Experts Do to Stay Younger and Live Longer

The facts, theories, regimens and suggestions we have been discussing in this book are applicable and beneficial to everyone. But it is also instructive to learn what the "experts" do to maintain their vigor, how certain people in sports, nutrition, medicine and other fields have kept their health, youth and vitality through the years.

When Don Drysdale broke the world's record by pitching his sixth shutout in a row for the Dodgers in 1967, it was an admirable though not a seemingly impossible feat. After all, he had the necessary skill and experience, he was in fine physical condition—and he was young.

But let's go back to the 1962 All-Star Game in Washington, D.C., and take a look at the man called baseball's slugging "elder statesman," Stan Musial. Sportswriter Leslie Lieber reported that during a crucial moment of that game, President John F. Kennedy leaned over and said to baseball commissioner Ford Frick, "I hope the old man gets a hit!" The "old man" did. A line single to right field. That year Stan Musial, at the age of forty-two, held more records than any other active player.

How did *he* do it, in competition with players twenty years his junior? Stan tells it like it is when he says, "The big secret about staying young is that you've got to work at it."

All the experts know that keeping weight down is one of the most important factors, and Stan is no exception. He thinks that this is also the factor that takes the most discipline, "like the will power to avoid overeating and reminding yourself ten times a day to hold your stomach muscles in. It alarms me if I'm overweight," he says, and he never touches greasy foods, gravies, rich sauces or desserts. His diet contains plenty of fresh vegetables, juices and lots of protein. According to him, "All baseball players are steak men."

Stan doesn't drink hard liquor but does follow the example set by Ty Cobb, who drank wine with his meals and advised him to do the same. Cobb "saw no harm in an apertif, even at the height of the season."

Stan's "cornerstone to keeping in shape," is exercise, eight hours sleep a night—and vitamins. "I believe in vitamins," he said, and proves it by his practice of taking what he calls "a bombshell of vitamins" every day.

It wasn't long after the All-Star Game that Stan retired as a ballplayer, but not from his job of keeping fit. The next job he took helped others do the same. In 1964 he accepted President Johnson's appointment as head of the government's physical fitness program.

Enos Slaughter is another major leaguer who, like Stan, was still an amazingly youthful and active player in his forties. A New York *Post* sportswriter, Leonard Shecter, described Enos as "the youngest 41-year-old man in the major leagues, and probably in the known civilized world."

In words just as enthusiastic as Stan's, though perhaps a bit less grammatical, Enos gave vitamins and a good diet credit for his reputation as "baseball's eternally youthful outfielder."

> Sunflower seeds [he said] and sunflower seed oil. I use a lot of

> that. I eat a lot of them seeds and we use the oil on salads and things like that there . . . And rose hips tea, I drink that. Got lots of vitamin C in it . . . and you gotta have a lot of vitamin C to keep goin'. 'Course you need B vitamins and all the others, and I take 'em all . . . I eat a lot of broiled food and stay away from the fried stuff.

Probably the champion vitamin taker of all time is J. I. Rodale, noted pioneer in nutrition. Author, editor and publisher of many important books and magazines on nutrition, health and physical fitness, Mr. Rodale gives a high-protein, low-carbohydrate diet, food supplements and exercise credit for the health and stamina he now enjoys in his middle sixties.

He is also convinced that they have saved his life. In a number of books and magazine articles, he has told of the heart condition he has had since childhood. Both he and his son, Robert, have reported instances in his adult life that triggered serious heart disturbances. They agree that any of these incidents could have resulted in the senior Rodale's death from a heart attack, except for two things: *His habit of taking long, daily walks, and the fact that he was well-fortified with vitamin E and other nutrients that protect the heart and aid in keeping the arteries unclogged.*

Mr. Rodale is a long-time crusader against white sugar, white flour and all refined, processed foods. His diet is essentially the same as the one endorsed in this book, which both he and I have written about and followed personally for years. But because his requirement for some vitamins is higher than the average, Mr. Rodale supplements an excellent, balanced diet of natural foods with a larger daily quota of vitamins and minerals than the average person would consider necessary. His reply to visitors who comment on the array of tablets and capsules is that they are concentrated nourishment and food substances, not pills. He makes it clear that he takes them to *prevent* disease by building up his body's defenses and maintaining a state of health that would be impossible without them.

In about the same age group as Mr. Rodale is former Olympic

swimming champion Bob Hoffman, author of many books, including *Old Age Is a Slow Starvation,* which puts the major blame for aging on a protein deficiency. Bob's physical activity and his nutritional way of life have kept him vigorous and youthful in appearance, attitude, and actions.

A common complaint among men and women in their middle years is, "But I'm getting old–I'm forty-five . . . or fifty . . . or sixty-five." Bob has no such sense of age and defeatism. "But I'm still a young man–*only* seventy!" he says. He *thinks* young and is a good example of what a cardiologist meant when he said, "Staying young in heart and mind helps keep the arteries young."

A Russian prince, Serge Obolensky, has had amazing success in maintaining his youthful looks and energy. Born in 1890, Prince Obolensky fought in the Russian revolution, and after escaping to England, lived there until he came to America in 1929. During World War II he served in the United States Army, and since that time prefers to be called Colonel Obolensky instead of Prince. Now head of a public relations firm in New York, which has as its clients some of the world's great hotels with internationally famous chefs, Colonel Obolensky still avoids rich foods. "My taste in food leads me, by preference, to a diet high in protein and low in carbohydrates," he says. "I avoid pastry of all kinds . . . For dessert I am partial to fresh fruit."

One of his favorite breakfasts consists of yogurt, fresh fruit or a large glass of fresh grapefruit juice and decaffeinated coffee. His luncheon may start with a cup of clear consommé, and it always includes a leafy green salad with an oil dressing. For a main course, his usual choice is one of these three: a broiled hamburger steak, lamb chops or seafood. For dinner, he has lightly cooked fresh vegetables and roast meat. His preference is for beef, but other favorites are roast lamb and chicken. A dessert of fresh fruit completes his simple but highly nutritious meal.

"I consider exercise of great importance in keeping my health," he says. Each morning he has a regular session of yoga "as a sort of setting-up exercise" and to keep him free of tension.

For more vigorous exercise he favors tennis and is an excellent player. He also plays golf, "for a few hours of fresh air and walking."

The colonel also gives credit to plenty of rest for his health and vitality. He has developed the ability to catch a ten-minute catnap almost anywhere, whenever he has the chance. "And each afternoon," he says, "unless I have an unavoidable engagement, I change into my pajamas for an hour or so in bed. At night I try to get eight hours of sleep."

His exemplary habits of eating, combined with a balance of exercise and rest, have kept his body strong, trim and erect, his face firm and unlined.

In other books, I have told how a number of Hollywood stars keep their youth and beauty. Here, for the benefit of my women readers, I shall single out "fair lady" Julie Andrews. She does regular breathing exercises before an open window and says that she "manages to avoid overeating, laziness and oversleeping." When she vacations in England, she admits that she can't resist joining friends in snacks of cheddar cheese, sliced bread and a quaff of beer. "But back in New York or Hollywood," she says, "there is no such temptation, and I am careful of my diet. I avoid fatty foods, all pastries and chocolates."

Julie says that she feels any woman can stay slim, attractive and youthful if she:

1. *Doesn't stuff herself,*
2. *Eats plenty of fresh fruits,*
3. *Walks as much as possible instead of riding,*
4. *"Saves her pennies on sweets and spends them on steaks."*

Her further advice is to "read some good books on nutrition—then do as they tell you!"

What about the nutritionists themselves? Do the men and women who write the books and give the lectures on nutrition follow their own advice? The majority of them do—at least *most* of the time, and it's what you do most of the time that really counts!

One of the best known is Harvard's Dr. Frederick Stare, who has been described as "lean, Yankee-rigged, a man who looks as though he has always been and always will be in his mid-forties." Dr. Stare stays lean, "Yankee-rigged" and looking more than ten years younger than his fifty-seven years by preserving his health and controlling his weight (and cholesterol!) with daily brisk walks, tennis, and a diet high in essential nutrients but low in total calories—*especially animal fats.*

"I am happy to see that walking is again becoming a respectable pastime," he says. "The idea is gradually permeating the national consciousness that too much sitting down and lying down are just about the worst things that the older person can do." Dr. Stare believes that most mature persons need more fruits and vegetables than they were brought up to eat. He recommends at least two servings of fresh fruits and vegetables a day, along with two or more servings of lean meat, fish, poultry or low-fat cheese, "and some liver occasionally."

Since all the experts agree on the fundamental principles of nutrition, let's see how they feel about specific foods. To a man, they are all weight watchers, aware of the danger of any food that is excessively high in animal fats and overloaded with calories.

But while many nutritionists will politely nibble at lobster Newburg or other rich, creamed food served them at banquets, there is one who bluntly refuses them. He is Dr. Jean Mayer, Harvard professor and author of more than 300 scientific papers on diet, who gives this explanation: "I'm a professor of nutrition, so I can afford to be rude. If I refuse such food, I'm doing my job." Of desserts Dr. Mayer says, *"I avoid them like the plague!"*

Dr. Ancel Keys of the University of Minnesota has made many valuable contributions to nutrition. In one of my earlier books written almost twenty years ago, I quoted him as one of the first to say that the number one killer of American men, heart and artery disease, was due to their high consumption of animal fats. It took more than a few years for *all* the experts to agree on the importance of keeping total caloric intake at a normal level and of drastically reducing the quantity of animal fats in the diet.

Reporting on Dr. Keys' "candlelight dinners," which are

famous among gourmets and his nutrition-conscious colleagues, Peter and Barbara Wyden told of his sample menu: "Beef broth pastini, boiled beef *without a trace of visible fat* [my italics], egg-plant with tomato and green peppers, fresh fruit and a flawless bottle of wine." With a relaxing highball before dinner, Mrs. Keys served what her delighted guests said tasted like "an excellent Roquefort cheese dip." She had made it of low-calorie, dry-curd cottage cheese, mixed in the blender with just a bit of Roquefort for flavor, nonfat milk, onion juice and minced clams.

Most of the experts favor the "educated nibble" between meals to prevent the hunger pangs that result in overeating. Dr. Keys is no exception. But he makes sure that it *is* a nutritional nibble by keeping two small plastic boxes handy, one filled with almonds and the other with dried apricots.

Adelle Davis is a human dynamo who has successfully combined six lives in one as a wife, mother, homemaker, lecturer, writer and consulting nutritionist. She has planned restorative diets for more than 20,000 persons suffering from almost every known type of ailment. The successful results she has obtained are impressive. And her vitality seems inexhaustible.

How does she do it? When she knows there is a stress-filled day ahead of her, she makes a point of eating a healthy portion of broiled liver for breakfast. All the organ meats are high on her preferred list, and iron-rich kidneys cooked in Creole sauce is one of her favorite foods. So is yogurt (she makes it herself) topped with fresh fruit, which may appear for breakfast, luncheon, or as a dinner dessert.

If she eats bread at all, it is usually when she has made it herself of whole grain flour and such real enrichments as wheat germ and soybean or peanut flour added to it. The only butter she allows on her table is blended half and half with liquid vegetable oils. The same oils are used for cooking and salad dressings. For a between-meal energy pickup, she may have a combination of brewer's yeast and calcium lactate dissolved in tomato or vegetable juice. (She adds calcium lactate to help balance the calcium-phosphorus ratio, since brewer's yeast is high in phosphorus.)

Knowing as they do that liver and yeast contain more essential nutrients than other single foods, the majority of nutritionists would agree with Adelle's statement that "Perhaps the fountain of youth is to be found after all in liver and yeast."

Nutritionist and lecturer Catharyn Elwood manages to stay "looking and feeling like a million" by a combination of sound nutrition and living habits that include adequate sleep and rest, plenty of exercise, and a wholesome, optimistic outlook. She shares the opinion of all the experts that "there can be no really buoyant health without exercise." Brisk walks are a part of her daily schedule, and so are some of the stretching, tensing, twisting and relaxing routines described in Chapter 12 of this book. "The ability to relax completely," she says, "keeps you refreshed and youthful beyond your years."

If her busy schedule permits, she, like Adelle Davis, prefers to make her own dark, highly nutritious bread and batches of yogurt, finding them both "easy to make—and fun!" Experience has taught her that the so-called minimum daily requirement of vitamins and minerals recommended by the National Research Council is far too low and that, for optimum health, the amount of each should be greatly increased.

We have seen that besides nutrition and exercise, mental and emotional attitudes are determining factors in staying young and living longer. Catharyn is blessed with at least three of these essential factors: an unfailing sense of humor, love of humanity, and peace of mind.

Linda Clark, the next expert on our list, is not a nutritionist, but a tireless reporter who has made nutritional research her life's work. According to her own report some time ago (never mind just when!), she was "pushing sixty." But what a youthful, vibrant "pushing sixty" she was! Her face was smooth and unlined. There was no trace of gray in her dark, luxuriant hair. Time had left only a gossamer touch.

Linda prefers to eat at home, because she says she can control the ingredients used in her own kitchen. She has two principles that guide her selection and preparation of food:

1. "Keep it simple but nutritious."

2. She follows the advice of Dr. Edward McCollum, who said: "Eat only food that rots, spoils or decays, but eat it before it does." Processed packaged foods with a long shelf life have no place in her kitchen, although she says that she "uses certain shortcuts which do *not* shortchange my family's health." Making yogurt is one of them, which requires "only five minutes to make twelve containers." Sprouting her own seeds and grains is another, which she says takes so little effort that she "could hardly time it on a stopwatch."

The meals that she calls "unbelievably simple" and easy to prepare consist of quickly broiled meat, fish or poultry "without sauces, gravies or stuffings," and large mixed salads of raw vegetables. To be sure of getting fresh vegetable oils and other ingredients, she likes to make several varieties of salad dressing every week or two. "I do not waste time on fancy desserts," Linda says, and she serves her family a choice of fresh fruit or cheese. The time she spends preparing nutritious foods is very little compared with the big health dividends it pays, and as a result, she says, "I find that I have more energy and can actually accomplish more."

Dr. Alfred J. Cantor has been called "one of the brightest stars in the medical profession today." An honor graduate of the Syracuse University College of Medicine, he is now director of the Sanford Institute, Flushing, New York. In his book on nutrition Dr. Cantor tells how he cheated death and regained his health by a change in his nutritional habits. Many years earlier he had suffered from intermittent claudication (narrowed or blocked arteries in the legs that restrict the flow of blood and cause a painful cramp or spasm). When he gave up smoking, his condition improved, but still no cure was effected.

Some years later he suffered a much more serious type of spasm—an attack of angina pectoris. At that time he was sixty pounds overweight. "I not only loved foods prepared with rich, fatty, creamy sauces," he admits, "but I would eat large quantities." Looking back on his dangerous eating habits, he quotes a French proverb, "Death enters through the mouth." He reminds us that we "dig our own graves" when we eat rich desserts, gobble candy bars, pour cream in our coffee or eat meats loaded with fat.

He searched for and found his own treatment, without drugs, for the atherosclerotic condition that threatened his life. By a change in dietary habits, he was able to reverse the disease. He put himself on a diet high in protein and low in fats and starches. Gradually he reduced the portions until he was eating about half the amount he had once consumed. Because he had a strong motivation, he *stayed* on the diet, determined to regain his normal weight. "I wanted to live!" he said. And what motivation can be stronger than that!

He discovered what he says has been "a life-saving drink." He calls it the Cantor cocktail, and he drinks it before each meal, giving it credit for prolonging his own life and that of many of his patients. There are several variations of it, and he suggests that you choose the one that suits your taste, or make up your own combination. The "life-saving" part of the Cantor cocktail is *one ounce of safflower oil.* Dr. Cantor gives the following proportions for what he calls "a one-two-three formula" for the cocktail preferred by many of his patients:

CANTOR COCKTAIL

1 ounce safflower oil
2 ounces of skimmed milk (fresh or reconstituted)
3 ounces of low-calorie soda

To avoid an oily taste, mix it in a blender or shake it thoroughly in a jar.

To his own formula, he adds an ounce of wheat germ and a 200-unit capsule of vitamin E, which dissolves in the blender. The exact formula doesn't matter, *as long as it contains the ounce of safflower oil and is taken regularly.* My own recommendation would be to omit any kind of soda, artificially sweetened or not, and use skim milk and fruit or vegetable juice instead. Or you may prefer to mix the safflower oil in a salad dressing, and use it on a large green salad twice a day. But if you don't use it that way, by all means take it in liquids, blend it with butter and spreads, use it in cooking—or take it by the spoonful, if necessary, to get your daily quota.

Other suggestions included in Dr. Cantor's longevity diet, which he still follows faithfully, are these:

Add ocean fish to your daily menu, "especially the readily available and inexpensive sardines and herring." (Remember that they are good sources of vanadium and other minerals—also of unsaturated fats.)

Forget about sugar, keep all carbohydrates low, and omit all hydrogenated shortening, pork and pork products.

Dr. Cantor eats liver at least once or twice a week. His diet includes what we have already stressed as the "traditional virtues" and the foods recommended to protect the heart in Chapter 15. He also knows the value of exercise, and suggests as a variation of jogging or running in place, riding an imaginary bicycle. Today, with his health restored and his weight normal, his youthful appearance and vigor prove the effectiveness of sound nutrition in preserving good health and longer life.

In my own books and lectures I have been, in a general way, suggesting or strongly recommending certain habits of living to others. But through years of experiments and personal experience, I have learned what boosts *my* health and vitality—and what lowers it. There is nothing difficult about the program that keeps me in top physical condition and out of the psychological doldrums that engulf many men and women as they grow older. Anyone can follow it. Most of it has already been stressed—but it still deserves special emphasis as the foundation on which health, longevity, and a vigorous, youthful old age are built.

Nutrition: With a few exceptions, the diet that I recommend for others is exactly the way I eat every day of my life. (Since I believe in reinforcing even the best diet with certain food supplements, especially as we grow older, I have listed the ones I take in the next chapter, "Food Supplements for Your Second Forty Years.")

The only exceptions to my diet occur when I'm attending a banquet or when I'm a guest in someone's home. The sight of rich, heavy food swimming in gravy or cream sauce sometimes tempts me to turn my dinner plate upside-down. But unlike Dr. Mayer, I'd rather eat a few bites of what I'm served than hurt the feelings of a well-meaning hostess. An occasional mild dissipation isn't going to make invalids of us if our daily nutritional habits are sound. In the long run, what makes or breaks our health is our overall pattern of living and the type of food we continue to eat through the years. I enjoy a piece of pie or cake now and then as well as anyone. But even on those rare occasions, they are made according to recipes in my cookbook, with whole-grain flours, liquid vegetable oils for shortening, and sweetened with honey.

Whether I'm at home or traveling, my meals are chosen as much as possible from the following:

For each meal, I have one or more generous portions of high-protein foods. It may be eggs, broiled or roasted lean meat, poultry with the skin and its underlying fat removed, seafood, yogurt, kefir, buttermilk, cottage cheese or other low-fat cheese.

Breakfast always begins with fresh fruit, not juice, and often ends with it, as well. Broiled liver, lean lamb chops and meat patties are breakfast favorites that keep my energy high and my blood sugar at a normal level for hours. In addition, I may have an egg or a cup of yogurt and sometimes a small bowl of millet cereal.

If I have millet or other whole-grain cereal, I sprinkle two tablespoons of lecithin granules on it. (It has a pleasant, nutty flavor.) If not, I have, *without fail,* lecithin stirred in tomato or other vegetable juice during the day. I rarely eat bread, but if I do, it's made of whole grain.

Luncheon is usually a two-course meal consisting of a large leafy green salad with safflower oil and lemon juice, and broiled lean meat, fish or poultry. If I want anything more, it may be a slice of fresh melon, berries or fruit. My luncheon beverage is usually a glass of buttermilk or hot or iced herb tea. (Yes, I do drink coffee for breakfast—but no cream or sugar, thank you!)

On days when I can't get away from my office, I have fresh fruit or a tomato and a cup of yogurt or a can of salmon at my desk. For extra protein, I keep sunflower seeds and almonds or peanuts (raw or dry roasted) in my desk drawer.

Dinner may start with a cup of beef or vegetable broth or a glass of dry wine. If the weather is hot, the soup may be cold. Perhaps a jellied consommé, a cold Swedish fruit soup or a variation of *gazpacho,* the traditional Spanish cold vegetable soup. The main course is chosen from the protein foods already mentioned. It includes the usual large green salad, with several additional raw vegetables sliced or shredded into it, such as zucchini, summer squash, carrots, tomatoes, cucumbers, asparagus, turnips, broccoli, cauliflower, cabbage, or whatever taste and appetite dictate. A lightly steamed fresh vegetable or two may or may not be included.

If my day's calorie intake allows it, I sometimes have wild or brown rice or a small baked potato topped with yogurt and chopped chives. (No, I don't count calories, but I can easily estimate them, and I don't go overboard.) Dessert may be a sherbet made of frozen yogurt and fruit or the customary choice of fresh fruit or low-fat cheese or both. One of my favorites is *feta,* a delicious, low-fat cheese from Greece.

Exercise: No matter how busy I am, I find time for long, brisk walks, stretching exercises and jogging in place. If nothing else, I walk part way to the office and back, up and down flights of stairs instead of taking an elevator, and when traveling, from the hotel to my lecture and back. Walking is my favorite way of exploring a new city, finding a different restaurant and viewing the changing scenes, customs and faces in a strange country.

When a deadline keeps me at my desk for long hours, I don't just *sit* there; I get up and *pace.* Several times during the day, between pacing and thinking, I jog in place for two or three minutes before an open window. When a man tells me that he hasn't time to exercise, I know it's just an alibi. He can *find* time if he wants to, during the busiest day. I know, because I do, no matter how crowded my schedule is.

Interest, optimism and enthusiasm: These are attributes of youth. They will be discussed in the final chapter along with other qualities that keep you youthful.

If you work at something that absorbs your interest and keeps you so enthusiastic and optimistic that you never intend to retire, you're lucky. I am among these lucky ones. But if I weren't, I would look for and *find* something that held a challenge for the future instead of memories of the past. I would search until I found a second career, a hobby, a vocation—whatever would keep me busy, active and in the mainstream of life.

What you do is a choice you have to make yourself. But others who have kept their youthful interests or developed new ones can give you the incentive you need to start. When I *know* what my way of life has done to keep me as healthy, vigorous and active as I was at thirty (and I'm more than twice that now), I can do no less than say, "It's worked for me. It will do the same for you. *Why not try it?*"

In the next chapter, to help you in your good health regimen, is detailed information about the food supplements that enrich your diet by providing concentrated sources of much-needed nutrients.

17

Food Supplements for Your Second Forty Years

Nutrition scientists have known for some time that many people who eat three meals a day show symptoms of undernourishment ranging from mild to disabling. Undernourishment can occur because of insufficient nutrients in the food consumed, and decreased rate of metabolism and absorption (especially after forty). For these reasons, we will see in this chapter why it is important to include daily vitamin supplements in your regimen—no matter what your age or how nutritionally excellent your diet—and how aging can be significantly retarded by the intake of adequate amounts of vitamins and minerals.

A recent United States Department of Agriculture survey stated that "in the last decade our eating habits have taken a definite turn for the worse from the standpoint of nutritional values." The downturn was described as the first since the department started its surveys of the American diet in 1936. "Only half of the households sampled were found to be eating enough of the right foods to give a nutritionally 'good' diet . . ." *And one person in five, or twenty percent of our population, was "in peril" because of poor nutrition.* Families in the upper-income groups, as well as in the lowest, the survey revealed, were in the "nutritionally poor" category.

Dr. Fred Senti of the Agricultural Research Service said that, during the last decade, consumption of "sweet rolls, pastries and the like" rose by fourteen percent and "a category called soups and mixtures," including gravies, sauces and icings, went up twenty-seven percent. The nation's consumption of milk products declined ten percent, and consumption of vegetables and fruits dropped by nine percent. "In every region of the nation," the report continued, "calcium, vitamin A and vitamin C were the nutrients most frequently found short in the average diet."

Speaking of the report as a whole, Secretary Orville Freeman stated that "there has resulted a somewhat diverse shift in food habits and some change in national dietary levels. "From this we must conclude," he went on to say, "that many are making a poor choice—nutritionally—of our food abundance, and that to a large extent income does not determine good nutrition." What Mr. Freeman called "expanded and intensified nutrition education" that will teach people how to eat for optimum health is what we nutritionists have always been working for.

The Department of Agriculture's survey has shaken up a number of officials who had taken for granted the nation's nutritional health. A study recently published by the Department of Health, Education and Welfare showed that in the fourteen years from 1944 to 1958, the vitamins available in our food decreased to this extent:

The vitamin C content of the average diet decreased twenty-three percent. Vitamin A had a twenty-two-percent decline. Vitamin B_1 was down sixteen percent, in spite of the "enrichment" of bread (after the natural vitamins are milled out of the grain!). Although the drop was less drastic in other vitamins, it was enough for serious concern on all counts. Niacin (vitamin B_3), the "courage vitamin," which has been successfully used in treating and preventing nervous disorders and mental illness, among other conditions, was down eight percent, and riboflavin (vitamin B_2), sometimes called the youth vitamin, dropped six percent.

Based on all the above findings and the fact that the diet which is adequate for one person can cause severe deficiencies in another, it is important that *everybody* take food supplements. Ten years ago I might have taken a more optimistic view and said, "Almost everybody over forty—except those with perfect absorption."

What about children? If anyone has perfect body chemistry and 100 percent absorption, you'd think they do. Yet vitamins are an accepted part of a baby's formula. And another bombshell was dropped when the reports and recommendations concerning a national survey of children were published in the *American Journal of Clinical Nutrition,* coinciding with the Department of Agriculture's report.

A team of experts from the Bureau of Nutrition of the New York Department of Health, the Mount Sinai School of Medicine, and the New Jersey College of Medicine and Dentistry made a six-month survey and diagnoses of hundreds of fifth- and sixth-grade school children, all from schools having a school lunch program. *They found the diet, the state of health, the teeth, and the nutrient levels of the blood poor in 73.2 percent of the children.* As a result, they determined ". . . to stimulate public and voluntary agencies to initiate programs of nutrition education *and nutrient supplementation.*" (My italics)

Harvard professor Dr. N. Ethan Edgington had this to say on the same subject: "Can science today say that our hypothetically healthy, well-fed child would derive no benefit from a properly balanced vitamin supplement? Emphatically, science cannot . . ."

Recent government studies, years of experiments by nutrition scientists, and his own distinguished research, some of which was mentioned earlier in this book, prompted the University of Alabama's Dr. Emanuel Cheraskin to make this statement at the American Academy of Dental Medicine: *"Every man, woman and child in the United States ought to be taking vitamin supplements."* (My italics)

No matter how young you are, it isn't too early to start planning now to *stay* youthful for a long and vigorous lifetime. In an article entitled "How to Prolong the Prime of Life" Dr. Paul de Kruif said that vitamins were "potent chemicals that will help stretch out your span of productive vitality. We now know that the time to try to push back senility is before we're old in years," he continued. "Old age begins to sneak up on us even in our twenties. What we eat—while seemingly adequate—may mean the *premature* aging of many of us. But by using chemical knowledge now available, *this premature aging can be reversed.*" He gave as examples some of the spectacular cures of the great nutritional therapist, Dr. Tom Spies, whose prematurely aged, sick and feeble patients recovered and maintained their good health by the addition of large amounts of vitamins and concentrated food supplements to highly nutritious diets.

Even though they "are identical to those naturally present in our food," Dr. de Kruif also stresses the need for vitamin supplements:

> Even in the best diets, vitamins may exist only in borderline amounts; and some people, because of their inborn chemistry, require far more vitamins than others. As we grow older, the need of most of us for vitamins rises; we can't absorb or use them so well. So, a diet ample for one person may be deficient for another.

The need for vitamins that exists during childhood and early maturity is, for the reasons above, almost always intensified during our second forty years. Moreover, as the years pass, some of the body's functions slow down. Metabolism is one of them. By the time we're in our thirties, it starts a gradual countdown. We don't burn up calories as fast as we used to, so in the majority of middle-aged men and women, a steady weight gain begins.

Middle age has been called the time when a man's narrow waist and broad mind change places. An important rule, therefore, is to cut down on calories as you grow older. For each ten years between thirty-five and sixty-five, your calorie intake should be reduced about five percent. Unless you make the necessary changes in your eating habits during your second forty years, you are likely to be among the twenty-five percent who are overweight or dangerously obese. All available statistics show that these people age faster and die younger.

Yet although you need fewer calories, you need more nutrients. The solution is to omit the foods that are high in calories and low in nutrients and to supplement your diet with concentrated nutrients that are within your calorie budget.

A recent report from German researchers states that unless vitamin intake is *increased* as we grow older, the individual cells lose their energy potential so rapidly that aging is speeded up. Drs. F. H. Schulz and K. Kirsch of the Berlin Institute of Medicine began their experiments with a group of elderly persons by testing the protein values and iron levels of their blood. Both were found to be low. Then, with no other dietary changes, the doctors gave the group a comprehensive multivitamin supplement containing, among others, large amounts of B complex and vitamins A, C, D, E and rutin (a component of C complex, or the bioflavonoids). Within ten days, these aging patients showed a decided increase in energy and in their protein and iron levels—*with eighty-six percent of them showing values considered normal for young persons!* The improvement lasted as long as the patients were given the multivitamin supplement. When the supplementation was discontinued, energy and protein and iron values dropped to their former low levels.

To meet your special requirements, you may need a combination of those available in the four basic food groups and in vitamin and mineral tablets or capsules. You may be among the many who need supplements simply because you can't eat the bulk of food necessary to supply all the essential nutrients.

It takes a long time to arrive at a satisfactory daily requirement for the "average," "normal" or "typical" person—because he doesn't exist. Dr. Roger J. Williams, professor of chemistry at the University of Texas at Austin, has made individual metabolic patterns and nutritional individuality a large part of his his life's work, and he says, "Even the Food and Nutrition Board of the National Research Council has come around to the view that the recommended allowances they decide upon are only designed for the *hypothetical, perfectly well* 'reference' man, woman, or child." (My italics) "Individuals need nutritional help," Dr. Williams continues, "not only to overcome illnesses that have already developed, but what is even more important, to help them prevent illnesses from ever developing." He believes that to do this we have to study and understand what he calls the "pronenesses" of individuals, and not try to fit everyone into the "average" category. Any time that I am not aware of my personal "proneness" as far as vitamins and minerals are concerned, I take far more than the recommended daily requirement rather than risk a deficiency.

Each year biochemists and research scientists discover new facts about familiar nutrients and their relation to health and patterns of aging. A recent discovery in the relatively new science of radiation chemistry has prompted me to double my former liberal daily intake of vitamins C and E. In an article entitled "Where Old Age Begins" (*Nutrition Today,* 12:67) Dr. A. L. Tappel, professor of nutrition at the University of California at Davis, stated that by altering the food we eat we may change the body's vulnerability to the damage caused by "free radical intermediates" within the cells, damage that contributes to aging.

> To begin with, [says Dr. Tappel] aging of our bodies appears to be influenced by an intracellular tug of war going on between two factors acting upon a third: intensity and duration of radiation-like effects; polyunsaturated lipids upon which they act; *and the vitamin E available to protect them from excessive destruction.* (My italics)

In simplified terms, this means that the free radical intermediates that form within our cells under certain conditions are the agents that start the tissue catabolism (destructive metabolism) associated with old age. They go flying around within the cells on a violent and patternless rampage until they strike and seriously damage other molecules. But vitamin E protects the cells from what Dr. Tappel calls molecular havoc and destruction.

He found that "free radical damage isn't just an isolated incident; *it is occurring all the time in the body.* Perhaps the reason some people look older than their years is that they have been more vulnerable to this damage than those who don't show their age."

Dr. Tappel calls biologic antioxidants "the counterforce to aging that these substances represent." "The best-known antioxidant of all is vitamin E," he states and concludes that "if enough vitamin E is present, the radiation will have little effect." Dr. Tappel also recommends large amounts of vitamin C in the diet to retard such processes as cellular and collagen aging and other causes of aging already mentioned.

Before the advent of radiation science, nutritionists were aware of these destructive forces within the cells and of the need for an abundance of protein and of *all* the nutrients in maintaining cell and tissue health and integrity. Dr. Robert L. McCarrison has effectively summarized the essential functions of vitamins:

1. Without vitamins, the body starves. Health is dependent on their action in the body.

2. The amount of vitamins required depends on how well the body can use them. There is great individual difference.

3. Each vitamin plays a specific part in nutrition. But all the vitamins work as a team.

4. One vitamin cannot replace another, though its function may be hampered by the absence of another.

5. All vitamins are needed to maintain well-functioning glands and tissues.

6. All vitamins are necessary to maintain an orderly balance between destructive and constructive cellular processes. If this balance is disturbed, destruction sets in and cells deteriorate, or "grow old."

7. The greater the deprivation of vitamins, the more rapid the onset of symptoms resulting from the lack of vitamins.

8. Vitamins influence markedly the production of hormones in the body, aid the tissues in resisting infection, and act as spark plugs in the body.

9. Extreme lack of vitamins and proper food means rapid dissolution and death. Partial deprivation means slow dissolu-

tion and disease. This state of slow dissolution is commonly known as old age.

Most of those nutrients included in the program to stay young and live longer I have recommended many times before. Among them are the supplements used by Dr. Lester Morrison and Dr. Tom Spies in rehabilitating seemingly "hopeless cases," people who were chronically ill, feeble and prematurely old.

Dr. Spies made nutritional history when he was able to reverse severe physical, emotional and mental ailments in 893 patients at Hillman Hospital in Birmingham, Alabama, who were so feeble that they had been unable to work for years. A combination of highly nutritious diets and what Dr. Spies termed "the four essentials" for successful nutritional therapy restored them to health and enabled them to return to their former jobs.

DR. SPIES' FOUR DAILY ESSENTIALS
FOR REHABILITATION

120 to 150 grams of protein,
2 to 4 ounces (¼ or ½ cup) of brewer's yeast,
Liver, liver powder (desiccated liver) or liver extract,
Large amounts of additional vitamins and minerals.

(Except for the chronically ill and those showing symptoms of an extreme shortage of B vitamins and the multiple deficiencies that afflicted Dr. Spies' patients, the usual recommendation for brewer's yeast is from one to three tablespoons a day.)

Dr. Lester Morrison has produced what he calls "a striking and gratifying improvement in health levels and well-being" in his patients with a basic program similar to that of Dr. Spies. Dr. Morrison suggests starting with two *tea*spoons of brewer's yeast a day added to skim milk, cereal or wheat germ. As your taste becomes accustomed to it, you can gradually increase the amount to one or two tablespoons a day. In addition, Dr. Morrison added the following to his patients' daily diet, which he found "to be instrumental in lowering the cholesterol content of the blood and in reducing the amount of harmful blood fats":

2 to 4 tablespoons of lecithin granules,
B complex vitamins in the most potent form,

At least 25,000 units of vitamin A and 150 mg. of vitamin C,
2 tablespoons of safflower, soy or corn oil,
2 to 4 tablespoons of wheat germ,
2 tablespoons or 1 ounce of liver powder, which he calls "invaluable for good nutrition."

Dr. Morrison also suggests a nutritional Molotov cocktail that "acts like dynamite in producing energy and vigor." You make it by stirring one or two tablespoons each of brewer's yeast and liver powder into a glass of tomato or other vegetable juice. Since both liver powder and yeast have rather definite flavors, if you haven't tried them before, I would suggest starting with a teaspoon of each and working up to the larger amounts.

Other Nutrition-Booster Cocktails

To make better nutrition as pleasant as possible, following are a few delicious high-vitality drinks that will help boost your daily quota of protein, vitamins and minerals.

A senior citizen's club of Ithaca, New York, sponsored by Mrs. Clive McCay, the wife of Cornell University's famous nutritionist, developed a fortified milk drink that can be whipped up with or without a blender. Club members have found it so valuable an addition to their diet that they call it their Fountain of Youth. And it's popular with children and teen-agers, too!

"FOUNTAIN OF YOUTH" COCKTAIL

1 quart low-fat milk
½ cup powdered skim milk
½ cup brewer's yeast
1 can frozen orange juice (unsweetened)

Variation: If you have a blender that can handle firm solids, with only one addition to the above, you can make a C-complex cocktail that contains the bioflavonoids as well as vitamin C, protein, B vitamins, calcium and other important minerals. Here is what to do:

Thoroughly wash one lemon and dice it, peeling and all. (It's the peel and the white membrane inside it that is rich in bioflavonoids—and the same part of an orange is the next best source.) Add to it the formula above or to any variations of it. If desired, use honey or black molasses to sweeten.

The next cocktail is my own favorite, especially when I'm under pressure and need to keep my physical and mental energy at a high level.

LELORD KORDEL STAY-YOUNG COCKTAIL

(High in protein. Rich in B vitamins, iron, calcium and other minerals.)

2 cups skim milk, fresh or reconstituted
½ cup skim milk powder
1 cup yogurt
1 tbsp. desiccated liver
2 tbsp. safflower oil
2 tbsp. lecithin granules
¼ cup wheat germ
2 egg yolks
2 tbsp. blackstrap or Barbados molasses
3 to 4 tbsp. honey

Combine all ingredients and mix in blender. If you don't have a blender, shake the ingredients vigorously in a closed mason-type jar. For a thinner mixture, add more milk (or if you wish, some fruit juice). I have seen two cups a day of this power-packed cocktail change the tired, despondent, slow-thinking person into one who is vigorous, cheerful and mentally alert.

Now, let's see what all this adds up to in a summary of supplements for either your first or second forty years, and the pattern of living that will keep you young and vital for a long lifetime.

Your 10-Point Program to Stay Young and Live Longer

1. *Stay thin.* If you are already overweight, reduce to a reasonably normal weight.

2. Keep your diet *high* in protein, vitamins, minerals and enzymes (from raw fruits and vegetables). Keep it *low* in animal fats and calories. Bear in mind that with each decade of your later years you should eat five percent fewer calories, but that each one should carry its weight nutritionally. From thirty-five on, you simply can't *afford* the "empty calories" of rich desserts and other high sugar and starch foods.

3. Avoid these three, any of which will make you age faster and die younger: *overweight, overeating and undernourishment.*

4. Avoid processed foods and refined carbohydrates. Substitute the natural or "complex" carbohydrates of whole grains, fresh fruits and vegetables, and occasionally potatoes and dried legumes.

5. Instead of refined sugar, use honey, which is best for all sweetening purposes. But not too much of it if you're watching your weight. Black molasses, date and maple sugars are also good replacements for refined sugar. *Unrefined* raw sugar may also be used, but consider it a compromise.

6. Include a half pint of buttermilk or yogurt in your daily diet. The calcium content of sour milk products is more readily absorbed than that from other milk sources. Their lactic acid content promotes good digestion and aids the assimilation of protein and B vitamins. From middle age on, we should do all we can to keep our bones strong and healthy and prevent osteoporosis, the porous, fragile condition of bones that makes them easily broken. Calcium is the primary bone-hardening substance, assisted by protein, phosphorus, trace minerals and vitamins D and A. Vitamin C is another essential nutrient, as it influences many of the body processes that indirectly promote bone health and strength. When I am lecturing in countries where buttermilk, yogurt or skim milk is not available, I carry calcium lactate tablets with me and take two or three with a little water.

7. Supplements for your second forty years: Some of the following supplements are those used so successfully in the Berlin experiments and by Drs. Tom Spies and Lester G. Morrison. Most of them I use myself and have strongly endorsed for years.

Since no program for health and youth would be complete without them, they must be repeated in this summary:

Two to four tablespoons of lecithin granules. Among its many benefits it helps prevent the moisture loss and the shriveling dryness that result in a wrinkled, aging skin.

Two to four tablespoons of brewer's yeast or two to four tablespoons of wheat germ. (Take both or alternate them, depending on personal preference.)

250 mgs. or more of vitamin C.

25,000 units of vitamin A.

500 to 1,000 units of vitamin D, or an hour of sunshine daily. (Vitamin D is not abundant in everyday foods. Cod-liver or other fish-liver oils are the best sources.)

200 units or more of alpha tocopherol vitamin E. (If you have high blood pressure, start with 100 units and increase it gradually.)

Broiled liver, any kind, two or three times a week

and/or

One or two tablespoons of desiccated liver stirred into tomato or other vegetable juice. (Unless you include brewer's yeast, wheat germ or the above forms of liver in your diet, a potent B complex formula is necessary to supply the essential B vitamins.)

Kelp tablets or granules (for iodine)

or

Ocean fish several times a week—and don't forget the inexpensive sardines and herring for their zinc and vanadium content.

Two or more tablespoons of safflower, soy or other cold-pressed unsaturated oil.

8. Try to get the balance of sleep, rest, exercise and relaxation that your body requires.

9. Whatever your schedule, you know by now how important it is to get in one or more of the following: a brisk, daily walk, jogging (outdoors or in place), swimming, or bicycling on a real or imaginary bicycle.

10. Water—and *watermelon!*—are both important parts of good nutrition and are easily overlooked. We are approximately seventy percent water, and the daily losses must be replenished. If you live in a hard-water area, six to eight glasses of water a day will supply valuable minerals. Water prevents dehydration, combats excessive skin dryness, helps keep the system clean and free from harmful accumulations of waste, and improves overall health, including that of the pituitary gland, which, you remember, controls all other glandular functions.

Watermelon not only adds to the water level, but helps cleanse the kidneys—the body's "filtering plant."

Sodium-rich watermelon rind juice is of special value in arthritis and as a kidney flush. Although I don't need it for those reasons, I wash the discarded rinds, chop them and put them through an electric juice extractor to make a refreshing, delightfully flavored and healthful drink that all of us enjoy. Sometimes I add some honey and freeze the juice into a sherbet.

Try adding a spoonful of natural apple cider vinegar to a glass of water two or three times a day. Vinegar tends to clarify the water, and the tart flavor may encourage you to drink more of it. Vinegar is also a good source of potassium, and its natural ferments pinch-hit for hydrochloric acid, activate the flow of enzymes and aid digestion.

To the first-time reader, some of the foregoing may seem like a tiresome nuisance—to pay so much attention to one's body. But the more you do for it, the more you will get out of it! Being human, it is expected that you will do a lot of backsliding—there's no doubt about that! And it's doubtful that you'll follow every bit of advice given. But if you are aware of your responsibility to yourself, at least you'll make more of an effort. Sooner or later it will all become a way of life. By then you won't want to go back to the health-destroying, life-shortening habits that may at the moment seem so difficult to break.

As your nutrition quotient goes up, so will your desire to stay in the mainstream of life, instead of letting it pass you by. You'll marvel at your mental and physical alertness. The interests and enthusiasms of youth that may have slipped away from you will gradually return—and what's more, you'll be able to handle them. Surely all these benefits are worth the small amount of extra care your body requires.

18

Making Old Age Wait

"Age has nothing to do with the calendar. Age is simply the growth and ripening of body and mind." So said His Highness, Mir Mohammed Jamal Khan, the ruler of Hunza, a country that has been called the land of eternal youth. This country and its people have become a legend told and retold in books, articles, lectures, and perhaps best known through the book and motion picture *Lost Horizon.*

Many nutritionists, including myself, have written of the Hunza diet and natural way of life that have kept this people youthful and vigorous all their long and active lives. Some of their recipes are included in my cookbook. But there are other factors equally important in prolonging their youth and almost perfect mental and physical health for 90 to 100 years and more.

"We believe that life is divided into three periods," the Mir continued. "They are:

1. The young years
2. The middle years
3. The RICH years."

They consider the "rich" years the best period of all. Time increases their wisdom, understanding, judgment and tolerance, without robbing them of their strength, ability and desire to work. There is no retirement in Hunza. "The idleness of retirement is a much greater enemy to life than work," said the Mir. "Our people—even the men and women over ninety—continue to work on by choice. We choose to keep active until the day we die, and we do not think about growing old."

In his book *A New Life in Later Years,* Dr. Heinz Wöltereck says that *if there is a secret to prolonging life and staying young, that secret is work.* While some people look forward to retirement, the majority of those whose lives have been the richest and most fulfilled would agree with Dr. Wöltereck. They are the ones who, like the Hunzas, choose to go on working as long as they live.

Herbert Hoover was one of them. When he was eighty-six years old, he said, "I've always been able to find new jobs that proved infinitely more satisfying than sitting around . . . It's my philosophy that folks should never retire from all work. If they do, there's a good chance they will shrivel into a nuisance to all mankind!"

Another former President, who through his own determined efforts grew from a frail, sickly boy into an active and incredibly vigorous man, held the same opinion. "No man needs sympathy because he has to work, because he has a burden to carry," said Theodore Roosevelt. "Far and away the best prize that life offers is the chance to work hard at work worth doing." A few thousand years earlier the Greek philosopher Galen wrote: "Employment is nature's best physician and is essential to happiness . . ."

Women have also discovered that keeping busy is essential to happiness and long-lasting youth of mind and body. Two glamorous actresses tell how they created a new life with a second career when the old one reached an impasse. "It takes discipline not to have anxiety about entering into older age," says Mary Astor. "Get yourself a substitute for anxiety over the passing years—reach for outside interests!" And that's exactly what Mary did. She joined a sculpturing class and worked with such enthusiasm that she soon had her work exhibited. Searching for another outside interest, she began to study writing, and kept diligently at it until she wrote two successful books.

When the lovely Irene Dunne retired from acting, she, too, reached for outside interests—in a position with the United

Nations. Her advice to women is this: "Keep your spine flexible, as well as your point of view. There is nothing that will age you like a rigid mind and a rigid body. It's taboo to say or even think, 'I can't do this at my age.' There is something for every age."

There is indeed something for every age, if we take the trouble to find it. For some it may be a second career or a hobby for fun or profit. For others—and I consider them the lucky ones—it may be the continuation of their life's work, which they still find absorbing. Edith Hamilton was one of the second group. After a lifetime of distinguished writing, her famous volume *The Echo of Greece* was published in 1957. She was ninety years old at the time.

To summarize: next to physical, mental and emotional health, perhaps the deciding factors in making old age wait are these:

Your attitude toward work and retirement and what you do about them.

Your own thoughts on aging and your will to live.

A psychiatrist, Dr. Karl Murdock Bowman, offers an inspiring example of "the power of positive thinking." In 1921 Dr. Bowman became chief medical officer for the Boston Psychopathic Hospital and joined the faculties of the medical schools of Harvard and Boston universities. From that time on until he reached the age of retirement, his life was crowded with work, activity and study. He distinguished himself in at least a half dozen different medical careers. Recently a new job was offered him. It was rugged enough to challenge a far younger man, and he accepted it. At the age of seventy-five Dr. Bowman became the first director of mental health of the state of Alaska.

Another "positive thinker" was Carl Sandburg, who, when over eighty years old, matched wits with Milton Berle on the comedian's television show. Berle was supposed to say, "You know me—I'm a brash young man," and Sandburg's reply was to be, "You don't scare me—I'm a brash old man!"

Sandburg objected to his dialogue, saying, "No, I never use that expression, 'old man.' I've got a younger heart than the general run."

"I noticed that." Berle grinned, and he cut the line of dialogue.

The waste of human resources through compulsory retirement has long been a criticism of the system that forces people to stop working regardless of their qualifications. In "The Waste of the Aged," a New York *Times* article, Dr. Howard A. Rusk explored the problems of forced retirement through the example of veteran sportsman Satchel Paige, who returned to baseball when in his sixties.

Dr. Rusk spoke of Satchel Paige's decision as "at least one heartwarming item in the news" during a week of international tensions and sadness, and said:

> The turn of the page in the calendar to that magic sixty-fifth birthday does not really signify one's ability or inability. Because of our lack of understanding in meeting the aging problems squarely and logically, we are wasting our most precious human resource and that is wisdom. Wisdom only comes with experience and experience only comes with time.

Satchel Paige doesn't really know his age, so he isn't conditioned to consider it a handicap. "The midwife died, and all the books burned up," he says, but from all available evidence, he is in his early sixties. Dr. Rusk points out that although Satchel's muscle fibers are old, the pitching wisdom he has developed through the years makes him a formidable foe. "Everyone will be pulling for Satch whenever he takes the mound," Dr. Rusk continues, "for he will be pitching not only for his team but for senior citizens who want not just pension but an opportunity to be members of the community, to feel wanted and to have dignity."

How do *you* feel about your work? If you love it, you'll want to stay in there pitching as long as you can. But if you find it boring and exhausting—and the two are generally synonymous—you may want to follow the example of the man who said, "When I retire, I'm just going to sit around and do nothing—*and do it slowly.*"

But one of the frustrating things about doing nothing is that you never can tell when you've finished! The worldwide insurance company Lloyds of London has compiled some alarming facts about idleness. After a ten-year study, they found that men who retire early usually die within a few years of their retirement, while those who keep occupied live considerably longer. The reasons for this difference are not surprising. Having no purpose in life, nothing to do and nothing to look forward to hastens the deterioration of mind and body. Sitting around thinking of your aches and pains makes the old ones worse—and breeds new ones.

A man's retirement presents difficulties and problems of adjustment for his wife, too. Women have told me that having a man around the house and underfoot all day is physically and emotionally exhausting. Dr. John F. Briggs of St. Paul, Minnesota, has made an extensive study of the problem. He says that without a definite plan, a man's retirement can be *"M-U-R-D-E-R."* Here is the way he spells it out: (The extra comments are mine.)

M is for the husband's *maternal dependency.* Like a child, he often develops a dependency on his wife for assurance, solicitude, time and attention that should be unnecessary. After all, *she* hasn't retired from cooking and housekeeping! She still has work that keeps her busy, even if he hasn't.

U is for *usury,* or stealing his wife's time. She has been used to some privacy and a little personal freedom without a man around, even if it's only time to do her hair and nails without interruption or having a neighbor over for coffee.

R is for *remuneration,* and there's less of it than formerly, so expenses usually have to be cut. Money problems may cause arguments, outbursts of temper and hurt feelings—just as they do among young couples. One woman summed retirement up this way: "It's twice as much husband on half as much money."

D stands for the *depression* that occurs when a man—or a woman—feels useless and insecure. In some cases, Dr. Briggs says, it stands for problem *drinking* due to personality changes, maladjustments and frustrations brought about largely by retirement.

E is for *eroticism,* or the change in *love life*. As noted in the chapter on sexual vigor, many nutritional helps are available, but understanding and cooperation are necessary for both husband and wife.

R refers to *retirement recovery*. Retirement is a traumatic experience from which both husband and wife may suffer. Reaching out for new interests has already been suggested as an antidote, and so has an avocation or second career.

Dr. Peter J. Steincrohn considers an avocation or hobby so important that he paraphrased a famous quotation for a chapter title in one of his books on aging to read, "My Kingdom For a Hobbyhorse!"

Expert planners advise preparing for an avocation while you're still young. Choose something that you've always wanted to do, by all means. But unless you expect to be fairly prosperous as you grow older, it's a good idea to prepare for something that will also bring in extra money.

If you haven't any particular interests, skills or talents that you can sharpen up, your local library has hundreds of hobby books covering almost every conceivable subject for both men and women. And don't forget that a hobby started just for fun can turn into one for profit. A retired man I know who lives in a small town became a local weather expert. He began with two inexpensive items. First, he bought a book on weather forecasting. Then at an optical store he picked up a simple, inexpensive barometer and began his studies. In time he became so proficient that the local radio station asked him to give his regional weather forecasts following the general weather report. The whole town, including the farmers and businessmen who benefited most from his forecasts of local conditions, took pride in the fact that he often beat the experts. Farmers timed their planting by his predictions, and housewives scurried to get their washing off the line if he said it would rain.

Photography, ceramics, leatherworking, woodcrafts, and many other interests can grow from hobbies into profitable ventures. But a hobby should be something that you choose for yourself, something that you've always wanted to do. All of us, no matter how successful, have hopes that have never been fulfilled and dreams that reached a dead end because we were too busy or too lacking in confidence to give them a chance. Noel Coward once wrote a song called "Follow Your Secret Heart," and if you've never had an opportunity to try it, why not start now?

Some of the best hobbies require no equipment at all except the willingness to help others less fortunate. Hospitals, churches, schools and community, civic, fraternal and veterans' organizations all need volunteers on a part-time basis for entertainment projects, discussion groups and many different types of useful work. Veterans Administration hospitals welcome singers, musicians, actors, readers, comedians and all entertainers. Their famous Gray Ladies are volunteers. Other hospital work for women includes participation as social workers, and nurse's aides, who may do everything from consoling or amusing a sick child to writing letters for patients or reading aloud to them.

Helping those in need can turn empty hours into those that are full and satisfying, not only for the ones you help, but for yourself. It can banish loneliness and depression, uplift your spirits and give new meaning and purpose to your life.

Harvard's Dr. Dana L. Farnsworth, at the 110th annual meeting of the American Medical Association, said: "The great sickness of our age is aimlessness, boredom and lack of meaning and purpose in life." Hardest hit by this "great sickness" are mental and emotional health, which Dr. Farnsworth describes as "that state of mind in which people can carry on their activities with satisfaction to themselves, with some responsibility to others, and without making nuisances of themselves to large numbers of other people."

He reminds us that it's the nature of man to have feelings of isolation, rejection, fear, anxiety, inferiority, bitterness, and hostility that exaggerate the usual stresses of everyday living, and to endure them he says that we need to develop these three qualities:

1. A feeling of basic confidence in one's self and others.
2. A sense of competence.
3. A feeling that the whole situation is worthwhile.

If I had to name one single thing that would do the most to promote all of these qualities, it would be this: *accomplishment.* Accomplishment in *any* field is an antidote to aimlessness, a lack of confidence, and an inferiority and other aging complexes. Sharpen your old skills and talents or develop new ones. *Learn to do at least one thing well, one thing in which you can take pride.* It can be almost anything that interests you, from playing checkers to chamber music, from making birdhouses to building your own boat. You can plan a reading program that will make you an authority on your favorite author or subject, help you learn to make flies and lures for fishing, become a history buff, an amateur astronomer, or an expert on your family's genealogy.

Dr. Laurence Morehouse of UCLA names another quality essential to physical, mental and emotional health and youthfulness. It's called spirit. "The spirit builds its own body," he says. "If your spirit is slovenly and lazy, your body takes on the same characteristics. But if it is vital and adventurous, your body becomes the same way." Dr. Morehouse believes that physical and mental activity and a variety of interests are vital factors in feeling youthful and adventurous and in improving the quality of life at any age. "And don't lose your sense of humor or get in the habit of complaining," he advises.

A beautiful and talented girl who was a teen-ager not long ago herself has worked out her own mature philosophy of life that complainers and nuisances, both young and old, would do well to follow. Here is Nancy Sinatra's list of negative attitudes:

Seven Dangerous Pitfalls to Avoid

1. Depending on others for the solution to every problem. (Remember what Dr. Farnsworth said about a sense of competence.)
2. Wallowing in self-pity.
3. Copping out without a fight.
4. Passing the buck.
5. Assuming a defeatist attitude.

6. Being afraid of failing.
7. Being stubborn and resistant to suggestion.

Whether you're a teen-ager or a grandparent, spirit, a sense of competence and accomplishment can keep you from getting bogged down in these emotional quicksands. Just as an adventurous spirit can keep you young, so can the seven pitfalls and a lack of purpose in life make you old and embittered, whatever your age.

Everyone is subject to occasional negative thoughts and emotions, and we justify them by giving real or imagined reasons for them. But we don't have to hold onto them until they become a part of us.

When novelist Booth Tarkington once asked a complaining, irascible companion why he was so angry with the world, the grouch answered, "A man's entitled to at least two good hates a year!"

"Possibly," Tarkington agreed. "But must each last six months?"

When you feel that the state of the world is all right to visit but you wouldn't want to live there, get angry about its condition—if you can make your anger constructive, instead of destructive. Whenever you can, substitute constructive thoughts and actions for defeatism, hostility, distrust and complaints. A change of attitude and a purpose in life may not alter the state of the world—at least not right away—but they will improve your state of mind. So whether you're young or old, let's start with that.

Consulting psychologist George Lawton, who specializes in problems of the aged, says that a surprising number of his clients are still in their thirties but "already worried by the specter of approaching age." "Your mind can keep you young," he tells all of his clients, from the youngest to the oldest. "Your mind is still young and growing at fifty," he says. "Your brain doesn't reach its zenith until ten years after that . . . At eighty you can be just as productive mentally as you were at thirty—and you should know a lot more." He calls his formula for staying young a youth elixir guaranteed to work.

"Concentrate on the part of you that's still young and growing —your mind," he advises. *"Keep your mind awake and active and you'll stay young all over . . . creative imagination is ageless."* (My italics)

Titian was still painting masterpieces at ninety-eight. Justice Oliver Wendell Holmes was writing Supreme Court decisions when he was ninety. Composers Charpentier and Sibelius were both hard at work past ninety. When he was eighty-four, Edison was busy in his laboratory. Goethe was eighty when he completed *Faust*. Also, at the same age Benjamin Franklin helped frame the American Constitution. Contemporary musicians who have lost none of their productivity and creative imagination include Pablo Casals, Leopold Stokowski and Igor Stravinsky. All are between eighty and ninety.

Picasso, the Ninth Decade was the title of an interview with the ageless artist when he was eighty-six. The preface described Picasso in these words: "The Master indomitable, with strength and youth everlasting."

"As with any artist," Picasso told his interviewer, "my past experience pushes me to work everlastingly more." His eyes held the enthusiasm of a boy when he said, "In sculpture, there is combat with the raw material. When I triumph over such odds, I feel the joy of an athlete after a feat demanding strength, muscle and cleverness."

As the attractive interviewer left Picasso, her farewell was "Good-bye, Master."

With his irreverent humor Picasso answered, "How I would like to say, 'Good-bye, my mistress'!"

You may think that these are exceptional men with exceptional talents. Yet Grandma Moses had never shown any particular creative imagination until she began painting primitives at the age of seventy-nine. From then on until she was ninety, her latent ability developed by observation, discipline and work. All her life she had instinctively followed the advice of A. J. Cronin, professor emeritus of physiology at the University of Chicago, on how to live longer: "Work, work, work, from diaper days until death."

Almost any parent or grandparent knows enough children's sayings to write a book of them. One grandfather did it. Art Linkletter's book about his television "family," *Kids Say the Darndest Things,* became world famous. I know a grandmother of five who thinks she has no creative imagination. Yet she dramatizes and writes amusing, exciting stories of her childhood for her five grandchildren. She has never tried to sell them, but they delight her family and friends, sharpen her imagination and writing skill and keep her busy thinking up new incidents to weave into stories.

Stanford University's "redoubtable" Dr. Lilien J. Martin had a wide range of absorbing interests and enthusiasms that kept her busy, and youthful, after she retired from teaching. At sixty-five she decided to learn to type. At sixty-eight she took a boat trip up the Amazon. She had never driven a car, but when she told herself, "If I'm ever going to, why not now?" she learned to drive—at the age of seventy-seven.

Discipline, a cheerful outlook and an adventurous spirit were the key words in an article written by Sophie Kerr when she was almost eighty. She spoke of the morbidly serious quality acquired by so many persons as they grow older, and while admitting that there may be plenty of reasons for morbidity, she concluded: You can't avoid growing older—but you don't have to be grim about it. Describing two women in their eighties as wonderful exponents of a fine design for old age, she said:

> In neither was there a scrap of grimness; they both were admirably self-disciplined. Neither complained, though both had plenty to complain about. They kept discussion of bodily failings for their doctor, dentist and oculist. Neither did these ladies talk wistfully about the past nor rail against the customs of the present. Instead, they welcomed change and innovation and watched with real exhilaration the speeding of progress.

Year by year we are becoming an older nation, an older world. And in some ways, a wiser one. Recently Dr. Edward J. Stieglitz, a noted gerontologist, gave these views on hope for the future: "Only the mature can reveal the full breadth and depth of man's experience. If we have an older population in the future, we may have world peace."

The national figures hold the promise of a longer life (and, hopefully, a more peaceful world) for the population as a whole. But what about you, as an individual? What will *you* be doing when you reach the age of some of the people who stayed youthful all of their lives? Will you still be in the prime of life at the age of eighty—or will it be behind you?

"At 80, we should not even be entering the prime of life." (My italics) This statement is the studied conclusion reached by authorities on aging at a recent Berne Medical Congress. "Living to two hundred will come later," said Professor Hans Schielber of the Munich Clinic, "but first we want to make man fit enough to go to work at eighty or even ninety."

A London dietician and consultant, Dr. Douglas Latto, spoke of all the resources of chemistry, biochemistry, nutrition and psychology that can now enable man to reach his full span of life. "We can live long," Dr. Latto said, "without growing old."

These words flashed through my mind at a publisher's cocktail party celebrating a Book Fair week. Some of the guests were older writers whose names had been famous for years. Others were young and talented newcomers whose careers were just beginning. As I watched them I noticed that most of the group had a number of traits in common. Young or old, nearly all of them seemed to have a remarkable vitality of mind and body, an eagerness for life, an interest in people—and a quick response to challenging ideas.

Someone introduced me to a charming woman named Emily Allen. Whatever her calendar age was, her mind and spirit were so youthful that she was at home in any age group. As I searched for reasons to explain her ageless quality beyond the obvious ones of excellent mental and physical health, I began to see a pattern. Whether it was instinctive or had been cultivated, she had done what psychiatrists recommend as an antidote for loneliness and self-pity: she had "crossed her life with other lives." Later my host told me that when Emily retired at sixty-five, she immediately opened her own bookshop. For the past fifteen years her interest in her work and in people had kept her involved with life and living. At eighty, her enjoyment of life and people was as spontaneous as a child's. She had the gift of drawing others out, and the ability to start a spirited discussion without monopolizing the conversation, as so many talkers tend to do. (If you're middle-aged or past, watch that growing—and boring!—tendency toward nonstop, repetitious chatter.)

We all age at different rates. As stated earlier in this book, each of us has three different ages. Our chronological age is marked by the calendar. Our physiological, or biological, age is told by the condition of the sum and parts of our body. Our psychological age depends upon how old we think, feel and act. The New York State joint legislative committee on aging problems has drawn up the following check list that can help you determine your psychological age.

YOU ARE NOT OLD UNLESS:

You feel old.

You feel you have learned all you need to learn.

You find yourself saying, "I'm too old for that."

You feel that tomorrow holds no promise.

You find no amusement in youth's fun, and their banter irks you.

You would rather talk than listen.

You long for the good old days, sure that they were the best.

You won't help your neighbors, friends or community.

You would rather win an argument than be right.

You have no plans for tomorrow.

One theory of aging explored by Dr. Alex Comfort and other gerontologists has been that our cells are programmed for living a certain length of time and die *when they run out of instructions*—just as a computer stops when it has done all it was asked to do. A Russian scientist, Professor Constantine Bykov, director of the famed Pavlov Institute near Stalingrad, cited evidence that the vital organs of human beings can be made to obey sound signals or other communications relayed to them from the outside. But until more research is done on the programming of cells and communicating with them and other vital organs, let's do all we can to keep them in good repair, and able to renew and rebuild themselves by giving them plenty of protein and other vitally important food elements.

Next to the program of sound nutrition and exercise that I have repeatedly stressed, here is a summary of the best ways I know of staying younger and living longer.

STAY YOUNG *by continuing to grow and change.* A few years ago, the distinguished painter, photographer and critic, Edward Steichen, said this:

"Change is growth. Change is living. I am now 82 years old—and still changing! I know that I am now more receptive, more keenly appreciative of life than I have ever been. All things seem fresher, seem newer to me, and more alive than ever before."

LIVE LONGER *by cultivating the will to live.* According to many doctors and scientists, people can live much longer than they think. "Unfortunately," says Dr. Peter Steincrohn, "they gear themselves for their exit at about sixty-five." "If we are really working at living," says Dr. Arnold A. Hutchnecker in *The Will to Live,* "we need not be afraid of dying. We can make every effort to develop our fullest capacity as human beings. We can strengthen every link that joins us to work, to other human beings, to the world around us. These are our safeguards against illness and against premature death. They are the deeper roots of our will to live."

STAY YOUNG *by keeping your sense of humor and the ability to laugh, if only at yourself.* "People with a sense of humor are ageless," says comedian Joey Bishop. ". . . The people I consider young are those who have found humor in adversity as well as success."

By keeping courage and hope in your heart, faith in yourself and others,

An adventurous spirit, a receptive mind and an unconquerable interest in life.

The great Belgian writer Maurice Maeterlinck said that at the age of sixty his mind seemed to have lost its alertness, its interest in new ideas and its capacity for work. "I shuddered," he said, "at facing unfamiliar things—people, scenes, ideas—a journey away from my safe, warm corner in the sun." But a chance meeting with an old man "who had never lost touch with childhood" resulted in a change of attitude that made him younger at seventy-eight than he had been at sixty. The old man had never permitted the years "to wither his mind, and therefore, in great part, they had spared his body."

Some years later, Maeterlinck wrote: "Today I am seventy-eight. Now, in my new determination and with that old man before me as a model, I welcomed all these, knowing that only by welcoming them could I live. I tried to touch life with all my senses, as the blind man illuminates his mind by the blessed touch of his fingers on the raised letters. *For belief in life, not fear of it, is the very essence of youth.*"

STAY YOUNG AND LIVE LONGER *by thinking of each day as a new beginning and by living it fully and finding enjoyment in it.*

A great heart surgeon tells of his vital sense of life:

> Express a sense of joy in being alive [says Dr. Michael de Bakey]. Bypass pettiness, and do something to make you feel good toward your fellow man . . . When I get up before dawn, there's a beautiful quiet everywhere. Night has washed the old day clean, and we have another beginning. It's magic. *A new start every day of our lives . . . to try something, do something.*

Science has already found many of the nutritional and psychological ways of slowing down aging, and you have learned some of the things you can do to make old age wait. Vladimir T. Kuprevich, a noted Russian scientist, reinforces our hopes for greatly extended life and youth: "I consider the aging process an abnormal process. I am sure we can find means for switching off the mechanism which makes cells age."

Today scientists all over the world are pooling their knowledge, their research and resources in an all-out effort which, in Dr. Kuprevich's words, is "leading to a revolution far greater in its potential significance than the atomic or hydrogen bomb . . . the conquest of man's age-old enemy . . . old age itself."

Index